MW00473024

If This is a Test, Have I Passed Yet?

Living With Inflammatory Bowel Disease

Ferne Sherkin-Langer

FERN
PUBLICATIONS

© copyright
Fern Publications 1992
P.O. Box 16893
St. Louis, Missouri
Ph: (314) 994-0052
Fax: (314) 994-0075

Macmillan Canada
Toronto, Ontario, Canada

Canadian Cataloguing in Publication Data

Sherkin-Langer, Ferne, 1955-
    If this is a test, have I passed yet? : living with inflammatory bowel disease

ISBN 0-7715-9046-6
Includes bibliographical references.
    1. Sherkin-Langer, Ferne, 1955-   .
2. Enteritis, Regional--Patients--Canada--
Biography.   3. Inflammatory bowel diseases--
Patients--Canada--Biography.   I. Title.

RC862.I53S54 1994   362.1'963447'0092   C94-900204-6

Macmillan Canada wishes to thank the Canada Council the Ontario Arts Council and the Ontario Ministry of Culture and Communications for supporting its publishing program.

Cover Design: Gary Stuber/Orbit

Macmillan Canada
A Division of Canada Publishing Corporation
Toronto, Canada

1 2 3 4 5   98 97 96 95 94
Printed in Canada

This book is dedicated to:

My parents, Ruth and Husky, who gave me life and then love.

My husband, Jack, who has loved me completely and has always believed in me.

My children, Jessica, Benjamin and Alexander, who love me unconditionally.

Thanks to . . .

There are so many people that have helped and believed in me and the need for this book. Husky Sherkin (Dad) for his financial support of the first edition. Alan Kerbel for his gift.

Denise Schon, Ann Nelles and Nicole de Montbrun at Macmillan Canada.

Jack Cole, Lenny Berger, Linda Scott and Gordon Cole at Coles the Book People, for the first edition.

Theresa (Doorly) O'Rourke at the CCFC and Terry Jennings at the CCFA.

Elizabeth Friar Williams who edited part of the manuscript.

Margaret Thompson at Thompson Printing who gave me wonderful suggestions and support.

Marilyn Finkelstein who helped me understand the parental side of the illness and co-wrote the chapter "A Mother's Perspective."

There are many doctors and nurses who have cared for me over the years. Dr. Kush Jeejeebhoy, Bernie Langer, Zane Cohen, Robin McLeod, Bryce Taylor, Jim Ostroff and more recently Michael Paul, who are jewels in the crown of medicine. Enterostomal therapists Diane Gard and Nancy Trepasso, who were outstanding.

Janis Shifrin, who inspired the title.

My family and friends who never gave up on me and continued to help me find the light on those dark days. Ryna Langer who continues to come to my bedside every sick day with a newspaper and an inspiring smile. My brothers: Bobby for his love and business sense, Kevin for his love and legal advice, and Michael for his love and "being Michael." My sisters- and brothers-in-law. Aunts and uncles: Lee and Mel, Chuvie and Teddy and Cindy. Karen. "The boys" and their "girls." Lynne, Ellen, Aviva, Donna, and Linda. DeeDee and Yoel, Fran, Angelo and Novella, and Laurie. Cindy, Janet, Lydia, Irwin and Annie, Andrea and Brian. Tom and Liz, Lisa, and Maxine.

The many sufferers, their family members and caretakers who have shared their stories with me, and who continue to be my inspiration.

And my husband Jack, who deserves special thanks for being my chief editor, computer wizard and creative director. Thanks hun.

Contents

Preface

Western medicine has to be commended for its emphasis on the application of science to the conquest of disease. In the past fifty years, we have made undreamed-of progress in the understanding and treatment of illnesses. Implicit in this process is the belief that science can conquer all diseases and that, if patients follow the prescribed course of action, they will be cured.

Our culture tends to deny that cases exist where our diagnostic techniques are fallible and the disease cannot be completely subjugated. In these situations, the medical attendants—including doctors and nurses—must not only provide first-class medical care, but must also guide the individual through a process of denial, anger and finally acceptance. Later, they have to allow the patient to control their destiny without endangering themselves. They need to educate the patient about the disease and the treatment options. Finally, the medical practitioners must be realistic and yet still give hope for the future.

This book is a graphic illustration of the medical establishment's difficulty in coping consistently and effectively with medical cases of this kind. The author, as a young person, had complaints that could not be diagnosed by "modern methods," and she was considered to have functional problems until her health was in crisis. The problem was that her doctor did not recognize that the results of so-called tests were wrong. Clearly, it isn't possible to conduct detailed, sophisticated investigations on all people with abdominal pain. But a major deficiency in our medical system is the inability to identify patients whose chronic symptoms need persistent review.

Later, the author describes being rushed from a comfortable and caring home into a hospital where she is subjected to painful procedures. She clearly requires these procedures to be saved from a very serious condition. However, her resentment results from the fact that she was not a partner in her treatment, but simply an object of the medical system practiced by her medical attendants. It is a truism that people will endure extremes if they recognize that it is for their benefit.

The need for control and for hope is a recurring theme in this book. These areas, not part of our medical curriculum, are pushed aside as we move towards a system of medicine that emphasizes procedures and potions.

Another aspect of the book is the window it provides on the courage, innovation and fortitude that people with inflammatory bowel disease must develop in order to prevent the disease from disrupting their lives. This insight is invaluable for anyone seeking a proper approach to such patients.

I believe this book should be read by all medical and nursing students as a real-life example of what is often taught in ethics, psychology and philosophy. Just as medicine cannot be taught without hands-on experience at the bedside, so too should ethics, psychology and philosophy be taught from real-life examples. An example becomes even more instructive when it is written by someone who is both a professional and a patient.

K.N. Jeejeebhoy M.D.
Toronto, Ontario

ONE

A Personal Note

I am a 38-year-old pediatric nurse with a wonderful husband, three young healthy, children (one girl and two
boys), a supportive family and loving friends. I also have
Crohn's disease. Today, life is pretty grand most of the
time, but it wasn't always so. Over the years, I've had
many hospitalizations, operations and crises. The pain
comes and goes, the drugs go up and down, and the
tests, discomforts and humiliations continue to engulf my
life for periods of time. This is the nature of chronic illness.
The details of individual experiences are different, but the
issues are always the same. Chronic illness is a constant
battle—a continuous challenge for the victim, family,
friends and care-givers. The challenge is to cope and survive with a life worth living.

The first time I witnessed my daughter trying to protect
me during a flare-up of my illness, I was sadly aware
the disease had prematurely robbed her of some of the
carefree existence that is owed a child. Instead of concerns

about taking turns or sharing with friends, my daughter's mind was often preoccupied with the fear that her mom might die and leave her alone. In the same way that my own mother's life had been changed by the daily worry about my health, the effects of my illness had infiltrated the next generation like a spreading cancer. Crohn's disease had invaded the lives of all the people I most cared for. It caused them pain, made them exhausted and worried, and did not relent.

Crohn's disease robbed me at times of my ability to show caring and nurturing in each of my roles as daughter, sister, nurse, friend, wife and mother. I was tormented. Later, I found others with similar plights. I have written this book for them—and for the people who share their lives.

I hope the story of my survival with Crohn's disease can help those who suffer the impact of chronic illness. I hope, too, that health professionals who read this book will be enlightened by the portrayal of the daily demands of chronic illness. These pages are filled with messages needed by anyone who comes in contact with people suffering from chronic illness. It has taken me a long time to reach the point where I can, for the most part, accept and cope with my disease. This does not mean that for me the work is done. For all sufferers the work of coping is never done—and that is exactly what chronic illness means.

People who are newly diagnosed often feel lost and desperate. Identifying with someone who has had a similar experience can help. It is easier to accept information and support from someone you know who has been through what you have suffered, and survived. These are the success stories that really count.

I hope to show how I and others like me can tap the potential to survive the ordeals we could never imagine possible. The search to answer the lonely question, "Why me?" will take readers on a long journey. They will find out things about victims of chronic illness that they may not have known before. Some of the information will disturb them. But I hope to present a new frame of reference in which to understand chronic illness and its victims.

Both new and seasoned sufferers may find a new philosophy of how to cope refreshing. It is also easy to allow the disease to take over our entire lives. Many of us cannot or will not share our experience because we are overwhelmed by negotiating our day-to-day distress. I hope to provide support and encouragement to the chronically ill to talk about their illness and how it affects them. Communication provides the freedom that is so important for survival.

In its mildest state, Crohn's disease—which most patients develop during adolescence or early adulthood—causes chronic diarrhea. Bathroom habits aren't generally an acceptable topic for social conversation, and trying to hide the need for continual trips to the toilet creates so much stress that some victims become prisoners in their own homes, terrorized by the shame of having an accident. Urgency and accidents create shame and guilt during a time of life when one's concerns should be about achieving intimacy. All-night parties with the main purpose of sharing deep dark secrets, first serious boyfriend-girlfriend relationships, experimenting with sex, are all situations that most adolescents must contend with. The risk of being "found out" may cause the Crohn's disease patient to back away from these normal challenges. Instead of feeling immortal, independent and increasingly in control of their destinies, victims feel the shame and anger associated with the loss of bowel control, something most people achieve at the age of two-and-a-half years old.

Talking to friends and family about something so unacceptable can be almost impossible. Young women, socialized to be attractive to the opposite sex, must struggle particularly hard to hide the disease's symptoms to avoid rejection. They are confronted daily with cramps, diarrhea and nausea. Instead of feeling good about their physical selves, they feel unappealing and may even feel self-disgust. Praise for being thin is about the only "positive" feedback a young woman receives for having Crohn's disease.

This book focuses on the difficulties of growing up as a woman with inflammatory bowel disease, and addresses the difficulties and incompatibilities of combining womanhood with chronic illness.

I often wonder how different my life would have been if I had not become sick. Even when we have a choice, we all wonder about paths not taken. In this case, the path was imposed on me as arbitrarily as if I had walked out on the street and been hit by a bus.

Everyone who collides with a chronic illness is obsessed by four key questions:
1) Am I going to die from this illness?
2) Why me?

3) Can I be cured and become healthy again?
4) How is this going to affect my everyday life, now and in the future?

Once we realize our lives are not in immediate danger, our thoughts turn to life as it was prior to The Diagnosis. We fear our future will be changed, but far worse is the knowledge that life will no longer be *normal*. Our lives are laden with uncertainty and the answers to our questions never seem to satisfy us. We become angry. No one likes the uncertainty that is and always will be an integral part of chronic illness; we all struggle without ever completely coming to terms with this fact, sometimes denying it, sometimes raging against it.

I have a cousin who has another kind of chronic, debilitating illness, which has evaded diagnosis for years. She suffers from an endless array of complications that intrude on her life without warning. She once turned to me during one of her hospitalizations and said simply: "I often look toward heaven and ask God, or whoever is in charge up there, 'If this is a test, have I passed yet?'" With a chronic illness, the answer will generally be a plaintive, futile "No."

Elizabeth Kubler-Ross, an expert on terminal illness, documented the stages that people pass through during the process of dying. By accepting the diagnosis of a chronic (though not necessarily fatal) illness, we are forced to recognize a fundamental change in our lives that can be debilitating, and sometimes even life-threatening. To a greater or lesser extent, we also pass through shock, denial, anger, the need to bargain and, finally, acceptance.

Although I had been sick for at least five years, I was nineteen when I first heard the name of my disease. I was still in shock when I was rolled towards the operating room for exploratory surgery. In the aftermath of surgery, my long-standing symptoms were pulled together and given a name: Crohn's disease. I wanted to cry and scream, and punch everyone in the room as they looked at me so calmly, or so it seemed to me. My breath started coming faster and my head felt as if it were going to burst. I felt the tears on my cheeks before I realized that I was crying. Questions flew into my mind, but confusion and terror rendered me incapable of speech. I wanted to stand up and yell: "See, you all doubted me. All this time I have had Crohn's disease." At the same time, I sensed a certain pleasure in having a label on which to pin my suffering. In shock, I was unsure what this awful, wonderful news meant.

How did I get from there to here? Yesterday, I was simply a person in a hospital room with belly pain and possible appendicitis. Today, I was The Crohn's Patient. I wanted yesterday back. I wanted to rewind the tape, to reshoot the final scene. I wanted my story to have a happy ending.

Left alone in my room, my denial intensified. My mind worked overtime. Didn't this white-coated messenger belong to the same profession of experts who had dismissed my stomachaches as psychosomatic? It dawned on me that there might be some other explanation, that this was some kind of cruel mistake. I knew they were wrong. I thought back to all the years that I had complained, and all the doctors who had shrugged their shoulders in resignation. Back then, it seemed everyone believed that I was making the whole thing up. I used to invent a multitude of excuses to explain the pain and diarrhea.

The medical profession had given up on me, and my family and friends accepted the opinion that I was well, and that it was time to "get on with my life." They could not imagine how much I wanted to feel well.

As I lay there, my heart started pounding furiously. I remembered feeling guilty and foolish about admitting that I had another stomachache, watching the raised eyebrows and surreptitious glances. I had felt that, by complaining, I was annoying the people around me. Each day, I had tried to ignore the gut-wrenching pain. Frantically seeking out the bathroom I was so dependent on, I wondered why I felt so awful. Now I was in a hospital bed grappling with a future filled with uncertainty, and consumed with the knowledge that my years of suffering had not been self-inflicted. Angry? You bet I was!

It didn't take long, however, for the anger to dissipate. Shutting my eyes tightly, I started to bargain with myself, and God. I ran through all the changes I would make in my life, if only the diagnosis would be reconsidered. A new doctor was summoned. I was convinced that he would deliver me from this sentence. But my bargaining went unheeded. Far from reversing the verdict, the second opinion was that I needed more surgery.

Many years later, after many more operations and battles, I can honestly say that I have reached a level of acceptance. Acceptance is the final goal, possible only through the development of coping mechanisms that do not accept defeat and that allow an individual to live life within the context of the illness and its unique, inevitable limitations.

Coping with chronic illness is not something you do once.

It is a continuous process, accomplished in different ways by different people. Coping means that you are actively engaged in adjusting and re-evaluating your activities and goals to attain the best quality of life available to you.

Coping can be viewed as a continuum: on one end is the person who has lost all hope, with the illness consuming their every moment and every thought; at the other end is the person who lives in complete harmony with the disease. Very few people fit either description; most of us can be found somewhere along this continuum. Our state of health at any point in time, the energy we can muster from our cache of inner strength, and the support we derive from loved ones and by sharing our story with each other all affect the place and the direction that we move along the continuum. Our goal must always be to inch closer toward the coping end.

In the chapters that follow, I hope you will find situations to identify with, stories to help retrieve your sense of humor, and some practical suggestions for moving along the continuum. Coping will make you a happier, more satisfied person, better prepared to get the most out of life.

TWO

In the Beginning

My episodes of illness always occurred in the summertime. While others looked forward to the summer, for me it would always be a season to dread. The first summer, I was only nine years old. At the time, I desperately wanted to go to overnight camp with my older brother. My mother had strong reservations about sending me. I was her only daughter and I was three-and-a-half years younger than my brother. She insisted that I was too young. "All my friends are going," I whined. Finally, Mom gave in, hoping that Bobby would be able to keep a big-brotherly eye on me. I was so excited, counting the days until camp would start.

After two weeks of swimming, hiking and nine-year-old homesickness, I came down with unbearable stomachaches, diarrhea and fever. Observing me in the camp infirmary for a few days, the doctor decided that I was not improving. I was sent home and hospitalized. Instead of camp food, I was fed by an intravenous line. Instead of lying in my bunk listening to ghost stories, I lay in a children's hospital listening to babies cry through the night. The diagnosis came back: typhoid fever. I can hardly remember the discomfort and diarrhea, but I know from my years of pediatric nursing how terrible this experience must have been. I was not grown up enough to read the fear and concern on my parents' faces.

After that summer, I often complained to my mother about my stomachaches. They would come and go. Like most adolescents, going to the doctor was an embarrassing experience. Thinking about discussing my diarrhea and pain with a strange man, and the anticipation of an invasive physical examination made the prospect completely unacceptable. Every June, my three brothers and I were trotted off to the pediatrician for our summer check-ups. The topic of my stomachaches always came up. I would never raise it, but at the end of the examination my mom would gently remind me to tell the doctor. I would sheepishly admit that I had been having "some trouble with my stomach." I was afraid that if I admitted to having a problem, the doctor would have to do *something* about it. The unknown *something* was my greatest fear. I resolved that it would be better just to put up with the treatment and hope that the pains would miraculously disappear. My doctor, who was a kind man with a busy office and crowded mind, listened and seemed concerned but was prepared to let things ride for another year.

The summer I was fourteen, I experienced my first bout of prolonged pain. It lasted for about two months. My mom, her face tight with concern, ushered me to the doctor, determined that something must be done. Now that I'm a mother myself, I can only imagine the frightening fantasies she must have faced. The doctor wanted me to have my first "GI series." I had no idea what a GI series was, and I was afraid to ask. The explanation I received was brief: I was told that in two weeks my stomach and intestines would be X-rayed in a clinic on the first floor of my doctor's medical building. Mom was to call for instrúctions about preparing me. Someone mentioned castor oil and not eating for a period of time before the test.

I left the doctor's office, my mind racing with a million questions. I spent the next two weeks waiting, preoccupied. I slept poorly, waking in the night and wrestling with adolescent nightmares. I worried that the test would be painful. (I was one of those kids who needed to be pulled out from under a chair when the doctor approached with a booster shot.) What about the results? What if something were really wrong with me? For the first time, I had to face that possibility. There was plenty of publicity in the newspapers about cancer. I couldn't consider that thought. I convinced myself that dying of cancer just did not happen to young people. Maybe I had an ulcer like my mom. I thought about her recounting the boring ulcer diets she had gone on, which consisted mostly of bread, water and an occasional cup of soup broth. Would I have to forego gravy and french fries in the cafeteria with my friends? I extracted as much information from my mother about the GI series as I could. She recounted her examination ten years earlier for an ulcer. She remembered drinking some "white stuff" and having X-rays taken. She did not elaborate and I did not push her for details. We were both terribly worried. We worried in silence. The day of the test arrived. I went to the radiology clinic and was told to change into one of those blue examination gowns that open in the back.

Feeling extremely uncomfortable, I walked down the hall toward the X-ray room. I was unaccustomed to parading around in pajamas in public. Once inside, I was asked to drink a thick foamy liquid which was called a barium "milkshake." It certainly was not like any milkshake I'd encountered: it tasted more like chalk than chocolate. I was told that the barium would improve visualization of my stomach and bowels. After a half hour of being coaxed, and a series of facial contortions that would make Marcel Marceau proud, I went out to sit in the waiting room until the "milkshake" had traveled along my gastrointestinal tract and the X-rays could be taken.

Two important things were established on that day that have stayed with me for my entire career as a patient, and which has shaped my career as a nurse. The first is how my disease continually challenges healthcare personnel. Whenever a patient presents the medical profession with a unique, *challenging* group of symptoms, they become "the interesting case." It is common for patients with Crohn's disease and other chronic illnesses difficult to diagnose to hear things like: "Wow, her gastric motility is so slow!" or "Come and look at this, Bob. It's incredible! We've never seen a patient take so long to digest the barium!"

I had to wait eight hours for complete X-rays. Each time they brought me back to the room to see how far the barium had traveled, I became increasingly discouraged. I kept thinking about how much effort I had made to drink it. I did not want to go through that again. What did they do to people whose bodies did not cooperate? They continued to marvel over what a unique case I was. The last thing in the world that an adolescent girl wants to hear is that she stands out in a crowd. Anything short of being a clone of her clique is practically life-threatening!

The second important insight I had was about my capacity for rebellion. As I child, I had always talked back to teachers and challenged my parents' rules. I had a mind of my own. My adolescence only increased my defiance. Over the years, this has provided me with a reservoir of tremendous energy for doing battle with my illness. But I also suspect that it has interfered with my ability to directly face investigative procedures and other aspects of the authoritarian medical system.

Defiance can also be a barrier to coping well. When the disease makes me feel sick, I respond with childish anger and defiance at the unfairness imposed upon me. I feel powerless. My choices are limited by the demands of the disease, as a child's choices are limited by the demands of her parents. Having to drink the barium that day made me defiant, made me search for a way around going through that experience again. I had to learn over many years that there were some things I simply could not avoid.

The result of the GI series was a suspected, but not clearly defined, duodenal ulcer. A bland diet was prescribed, some nebulous words of advice were given and life went on. In their usual fashion, the bellyaches subsided and both the diet and the awful day with the radiologist faded from memory.

During my seventeenth summer, my stomachaches worsened and I found myself popping Tylenol simply to keep up and participate in daily activities. I was admitted to the local children's hospital and met the first in a long line of gastroenterologists. Everyone in my family, myself included, responded with mixed feelings about inviting a "specialist" into our lives. For many families, a specialist represents another, more intense, invasion of privacy. There are the same endless questions and answers, and a new series of more embarrassing and uncomfortable examinations. The hardest part, however, is confronting the reality of a serious problem for the first time.

During this hospitalization, my age was a source of stress for me. I was one of the oldest patients in a facility that provided few resources for my emotional and physical needs. My privacy was assaulted on a daily basis. A chart recording all my bowel movements was conspicuously displayed on the wall facing everyone who entered my room. I became more and more embarrassed as my bowel habits became a major topic of conversation, no matter who came into my room. When I saw someone glance at the latest entry on the record, I wanted to disappear. I felt horribly uncomfortable and embarassed, and didn't want to think or talk about what might be wrong. Even after years of symptoms, part of me still wanted to believe that, if I did not talk about them, the symptoms would magically disappear.

On the first Saturday night of that hospitalization, my friends went to a Jethro Tull rock concert without me. I felt particularly bitter and my boyfriend was visibly upset as he said good-bye. I watched them all sneak down the back stairs because they had stayed past visiting hours. I cried hard as I walked back to my room. It was not fair: I was being deprived of something that was very important to me. Today, the thought of missing a rock concert seems trivial, but at the time it was a major disappointment in my life. Over the years, many others would follow.

That summer I had my first sigmoidoscopy—a procedure surely developed during the Spanish Inquisition. The test took place in a large, impressively equipped examining room. The sigmoidoscopy tube is about one-and-a-half inches in diameter and three feet long. Its main purpose is to visualize the tissue at the lower end of the large bowel. It is placed into the rectum and advanced until the doctor has had an adequate look at the bowel. Compared to this, chalk milkshakes seemed wonderful. I decided that this would be the last time I would undergo any of these horrendous procedures. (Little did I know what future horrors lay ahead and how powerless I would be to protect myself from them.)

After all the trauma and talking, the gastroenterologist reported with a smile that nothing abnormal had been found. I felt relieved and my whole family went out on the town to celebrate. With a false sense of hope, I resumed Tylenol-popping and my adolescent dreams.

The summer before my last year of high school, I went to France with my best friends. We felt so grown up and in charge of our destinies as we waved good-bye to our parents. As we boarded our last connection to Nice, in the south of France, Jane, Lynne, Pam and I made a pact to learn French, meet lots of new people and above all have the time of our lives. But intermittent diarrhea and sporadic episodes of rectal bleeding began two weeks after we arrived. I confided to Lynne about my stomachaches. She listened but as I saw her start to look worried, I felt that I was breaching our summer pact. I resolved not to give in to this "stuff" anymore. The natural optimism of adolescence, and the desire not to give up my wonderful summer with my best friends, helped support my denial. It became a challenge to learn what foods I could tolerate and the location of all bathrooms along the routes we frequented. I thought as little as possible about the danger signals, and tried to ignore my body's unreliability. This was not exactly the summer of fun I had promised myself.

Towards the end of the summer, I traveled to Switzerland with Lynne and her boyfriend. This part of our trip was to have lasted seven days but on the fourth day, amidst the beauty of Zurich, the illness struck with force. I was terrified and nearly hysterical when I looked into the toilet and saw blood. This had nothing to do with my period. With Lynne's help, I booked an airline ticket and phoned home, alerting my parents to the sudden change of plans. Lonely, frightened and feeling cheated, I waved good-bye to my friends: no one was laughing this time. On the flight home, I stared out the window, hoping no one would look directly at me. I was afraid I was going to cry. I breathed deeply to calm myself, closed my eyes and hoped that I could sleep away the time remaining until I was reunited with my parents.

Back home, wrapped in their protective arms, I felt safe. The contrast between the freedom of my European fling, and practically sitting on my mother's lap as I was taken to the doctor, was overwhelming. I felt angry at them, at myself and at my illness for pushing me backwards; holding me back from adulthood. I was so jealous of my friends in Europe but I was even more scared about my health and my future.

My doctor ordered some stool cultures and other non-invasive tests. No diagnosis was made, and the bleeding stopped. The doctors concluded that I'd picked up a parasite while in Europe but I no longer believed what they said. This time, I didn't want to celebrate with my family. I felt as if I were walking on eggshells, which at any time could break and reveal the whole mess beneath.

That fall, I entered a four-year nursing program at the University of Toronto to fulfill a lifelong ambition to be a nurse. My parents had always encouraged me to pursue my nursing education at the university level. Although my father was a successful businessman, he had had limited schooling. For my mother, a university education was not a consideration due to the size of her family: with a family of six girls and two boys, the university education was reserved for the boys. Like so many parents, mine wanted me to have the best education possible—to have the opportunities they never had. Crohn's disease came close to shattering our dreams.

During my entire first year at university, I was ill. I began first term with mononucleosis, which I had probably caught from my boyfriend Jack, who I'd met the previous summer. For four months I walked around the campus half-asleep, with a crew of tiny construction workers hammering and pounding in my head. In the spring, I had to complete a one-month block of bedside nursing at the local veteran's hospital. Each day, I felt sicker. Constant diarrhea compromised my ability to give my patients uninterrupted care. Numerous times I had to excuse myself, run from the room and find a bathroom.

Fortunately, there were no earth-shattering consequences (I was not practicing on acutely ill patients), but the experience did shatter my confidence. How could I achieve my professional goals if I had to deal constantly with my wretched bowels?

Over the course of a month, the pain and diarrhea gradually intensified. I became listless, run down and lost weight. I was tired and felt like I had no energy. Jack suggested that my ulcer might be acting up and, because I had read somewhere that it was good for ulcers, I began drinking milk in large quantities. I was so weak I did not even notice that the diarrhea and pain grew worse. (Much later, I found out that I had lactose intolerance, which causes severe diarrhea and pain when milk is consumed.)

The last day of my clinical rotation, I dragged myself to my final evaluation. I could not believe I had made it. After pushing my body to its limit; after all the nights staying up late to prepare for nursing my patients the following day; and after watching girls in my class drop out under the pressure, I had made it. It was almost as if the challenge of the undiagnosed illness made me fight harder. I received a top mark but, instead of being happy and amazed at my accomplishment, all I cared about was ridding myself of the huge responsibility school represented. I would no longer have to contend with a schedule that intensified the daily cycle of diarrhea, pain and embarrassment.

All that year, I had refused to see a doctor because I was afraid he would stop me from completing my first year of nursing school. I was also afraid that, if I lost the momentum and left school, I might never return. After my final evaluation, my mother drove me to the doctor's office. That drive was the beginning of the worst yet. Every small bump in the road caused a jolt of pain. Just breathing was excruciating. I felt cold and nauseated, and realized that I was losing track of time. My mother led me into the elevator and up to the doctor's office. He took one look at me, made a quick phone call, and packed me off to the hospital emergency room.

THREE

Adolescents Don't Have Bowels, So How Come I've Got Crohn's Disease?

The events that followed remain in my mind like shards of half-remembered images from a protracted nightmare. Some of the images are sharp; others, less so. It's clear, however, that this period of spiraling illness and surgery—as well as the awareness of my mortality—has affected me more than any other experience since.

One indelible image is of the intern who, shortly after I was admitted, put a nasogastric tube down one nostril and into my stomach. This was to stop me from vomiting the contents of my stomach during surgery. Impudent and insensitive, he seemed incapable of dealing compassionately with someone who was sick and frightened. He arrived in my room with a three-foot-long tube resting on a kidney-shaped dish of ice and announced that this monstrosity was going down my nose and into my stomach. Without further ado, he roughly cranked up my bed, sending waves of pain into my inflamed abdomen, and assaulted my nose with it. The tube felt uncomfortable at first, but I wasn't prepared for the sensation of not being able to breathe. As it passed by my gag reflex, the contents of my stomach emptied out my mouth and nose in a violent spasm of vomiting. I felt as if I was being smothered and began yanking at the tube. The intern's mission was thwarted as my final yank pulled it from my nostril. I was ecstatic to be rid of it and started to relax when, suddenly, the intern's attack changed from physical to verbal: "Do you realize what you've done?" he shouted. "You're such a goddamn baby! Now, lie back quietly because I have to do this, and you'd better cooperate."

My parents and Jack had been asked to wait outside. I was furious at them for allowing this inexperienced imbecile to invade my body like that. They were supposed to protect me, weren't they? I kept staring at the door expecting them to burst through and disarm the perpetrator. But no one came to my rescue and the tube finally went down. I lay exhausted from the fight, feeling violated and angry. "I hate you," I croaked at the intern as he left my room.

When I was transferred to a stretcher and wheeled through the doorway of my hospital room, I saw the looks of pain and helplessness on the faces of Jack and my parents. For a moment, as I was slowly wheeled past them towards the bank of service elevators, I hated them, too, for allowing my body to be assaulted. Had I lost all my rights and dignity as a human being?

Some hours later, after the surgery, I awoke with an oxygen mask on my face, feeling as if I had just come

in second in a prize fight. Drifting in and out of consciousness, I wondered why the nurses kept asking me
my name. Didn't they know who I was? Before I had
a chance to worry about it, I drifted away again.

During doctors' rounds the next morning, I finally learned
my diagnosis: Crohn's disease. It had a strange but sooth-
ing sound to it. I was told that Crohn's disease had sec-
ondarily caused my attack of appendicitis. My appendix
had been removed but my large bowel was severely inflamed from the disease. To help my bowels, I was receiving medication intravenously.

With this announcement, my illness seemed focused.
The enemy had a name: I now knew what I was fighting.
What I didn't realize was that the battle had just begun.

Crohn's disease is an inflammatory bowel disease that
is usually diagnosed in people in their late teens or early
twenties—although it can, and does, occur in young children or older adults. It is very unpredictable and affects
each person with a different intensity. Some people have
one "bout" and don't experience it again until twenty years
later. Some may never experience it twice. For others,
it hits hard and is relentless. Despite these variations in
intensity, it is a chronic, lifelong threat to everyone suffering from it.

The most common symptoms are severe diarrhea, persistent debilitating pain, fevers, weight loss, fatigue and
an inability to tolerate certain foods—especially fresh
fruits, vegetables and other high-fibre foods. Crohn's disease can attack, ulcerate and scar any of the tissue along
the entire gastrointestinal tract, from the mouth to the

anus, although it usually involves the small bowel and colon. Most affected individuals have at least one major operation, such as a bowel resection, to remove a piece of severely diseased bowel. Surgery doesn't cure the disease but it can help the patient when drug therapy fails or complications occur. Although it's unclear what causes Crohn's disease, the principal theory is that it is an auto-immune disease in which the body fails to recognize its own tissue. When this happens, the body's immune system attacks the tissue of the gastrointestinal tract, trying to destroy it as it would any invader.

The next ten days in the hospital were grim. Medication, on which we had pinned our hopes, didn't stop the course of the disease: my large bowel was slowly being destroyed by this relentless, newly defined enemy. The pain grew worse and the days longer. I slept less and less and dreaded night, with its hours of silent darkness, when it seemed everyone else in the world was sleeping. As the pain overwhelmed me, shutting out everything, I began to feel that I was losing the fight.

My abdomen filled with air and became more distended with each passing eight-hour shift of nurses. My pediatrician came to visit and percussed my abdomen. It was swollen like the bellies of famine-stricken children on TV advertisements. The pain medication was supposed to last for four hours, but its effects wore off after only one. Then the Infamous Intern decided that I must be addicted to the pain medication, and cut back the dose to every six hours. When I became hysterical, he seemed to smirk, and pointed to my hysteria as further evidence that I was on my way to becoming a crazed addict. I told him the pain was so bad I was sure I was going to die. I couldn't understand why he wouldn't make my death bed more comfortable. Since I would probably die from the pain, I reasoned, I could hardly become an addict. The last word, however, was his. "No way," he said, and turned on his heel for another infuriating grand exit.

People began examining me more often. When they asked me to move my body across the bed so that it would be easier to examine me, I cried from the pain. Even crying hurt. The young orderly who steered my wheelchair downstairs for X-rays must have spent his weekends driving cars in smash-up derbies. Each bump and jostle hurt—I could no longer remember the last time I had felt pain-free. The first set of X-rays were followed by a second set some hours later. The second ride down was even worse. When I got back to my room again, I was greeted by an ominous group of familiar but concerned faces. Jack and my parents were standing near my bed, waiting. Something was wrong!

FOUR

The Ileostomy

Your colon has to come out," said one doctor. "You have toxic megacolon," said another. "Colon—come out? Toxic what?" My mother, who can stay calm when necessary, intervened, and in a very authoritative voice asked for another opinion. Within half an hour, I received a visit from a prominent gastroenterologist who had extensive experience with Crohn's disease. Waiting for his arrival, I felt numb.

The gastroenterologist was a man of medium height with black hair and dark brown eyes behind heavy black-framed glasses. As he approached my bed, I saw the compassion in his face and realized that this was a person used to dealing with pain and suffering. After a quick assessment, he said: "You need your colon out, and you need an ileostomy." I searched his face, looking for clues as to what this meant. I was unsure what an ileostomy was but had a vague sense that it wasn't good. As he explained, I became horrified.

"Creation of an ileostomy requires taking a piece of your small bowel and bringing it out to the surface of your abdomen. This is called a stoma. Instead of having a bowel movement in the traditional way, a bag will be placed over the stoma. When it fills, you can empty it into the toilet the way you do now."

All I could visualize was a large trash bag. How was I going to tote it around? I mustered all my strength and, in my most condescending nineteen-year-old voice, said: "Well, what if I don't have the operation?" I suppose that I was trying to scare off the verdict by acting as if what he'd just said was completely ridiculous. He looked at me for a moment, and then calmly replied: "You'll die."

We have all, at one time or another, talked about dying of laughter or embarrassment, or wished that we would die rather than experience something unpleasant. My next thought was that I would rather die than have an ileostomy. I couldn't focus on the life-and-death seriousness of it. I was immediately obsessed with how this would alter my body. How could I possibly adjust? Would I ever wear a bikini again or feel comfortable enough to go skinny-dipping? Would my boyfriend want to hug and kiss me, knowing that I was wearing this bag on my abdomen? For the first time in ten days, my mind was free of pain as I struggled to deal with the implications of this surgery.

While I craved reassurance that my life wouldn't change, I saw from the looks on the faces surrounding my bed that other issues were more critical. My questions must have seemed trivial to them. They were concerned that I might not survive the next twenty-four hours and weren't giving much thought to the quality of my life, as seen through my adolescent eyes. But, critical or not,

I couldn't help being aware that the image I always had of myself had just been shattered.

For the impending surgery, I was transferred to another hospital through an underground tunnel. Jack helped push the stretcher as my terrified parents, left behind, alone and terrified, watched us disappear into the tunnel's darkness. I held tightly to Jack's hand while he steered me along. We talked about who he should call and what he should say to our mutual friends. We agreed on telling them that I was going to have more surgery and that no one would know exactly what needed to be done until the surgeon opened me up. I was satisfied with this story as I repeated our vow of silence regarding the ileostomy. "You aren't to tell anyone," I said over and over. "Not Lynne or Ellen or anyone." As the bumpy ride brought fresh waves of pain, I squeezed Jack's hand even tighter. I didn't care anymore what they did to me as long as I would feel relief from the pain and be able to get some sleep.

I woke up many hours later in the recovery room. I remembered little of what had happened. Most of the images in my mind were blurred. My first thought was that someone had driven a tractor-trailer up, down and sideways across my entire belly. I drifted again. When my head finally cleared, I looked up to see three strained, smiling faces poking out of protective white gowns. Relief was evident all over Mom, Dad and Jack's faces. I closed my eyes knowing that I was alive and safe, at least for now.

The Intensive Care Unit was another new experience, filled with machines that whirred, buzzed and beeped day and night. I was constantly being asked to do something.

Sometimes I was sticking out my skinny arms for the vampirish blood lady, who would walk away with her thirteen daily vials. Other times I was asked to lie still for blood pressure, temperature and pulse readings, or asked to move, breathe and cough, routines designed to inflict pain and prevent pneumonia. Too tired to mind all the fuss, I seemed to sleep through most of it. The narcotics and gentle and considerate nursing care kept me as comfortable as possible. The intense pain of the past ten days, like everything else, seemed all part of a bad dream from which I was slowly waking.

On my first walk down the hall, I was wired for sound. Everyone was in on the act. Mom held one arm, Dad held the other and poor Jack was assigned the unromantic task of pushing my IV pole, with tubes carrying the necessary fluids in and other tubes draining the bad stuff out of my healing body. My older brother Bobby followed along, spouting cheers and encouragement as we took each vital step. After the long odyssey to the end of the hallway and back, I settled into bed for a nap. Just as sleep overcame me, my gastroenterologist and his band of Merry Men announced their arrival. He discussed my "case" at great length with them. Although the information was about me, I felt as if I were eavesdropping. When he was finished talking, he looked down and ordered me to start moving, warning of the dangers of post-operative pneumonia if I didn't comply. With this decree, he and his entourage moved towards the door. Glaring at his receding back, I loudly informed him—and everyone else within a three-mile radius—that I had just returned from a long walk. He turned, looked at me and then, as if he had suddenly discovered there was a person inside my frail body, a smile appeared on his face. "Good job," he said, "keep up the good work."

The second day in the Intensive Care Unit, as my nurse was changing my abdominal bandages, I set eyes on my ileostomy for the first time. I had been uncertain what to expect, and was surprised at how small it was. My belly still looked like my belly, but there was a strange addition to it which looked somewhat like a rosebud. The nurse quietly informed me that this was my new stoma. I was still feeling so ill that I allowed the large bandages covering my abdomen to insulate me from dealing with this alteration in my basic anatomy. On the third day, a male nurse was assigned to look after me. I demanded that he be removed from my room immediately. He was a small man, and very pleasant, but I wasn't ready for any male other than my doctor to see my new body. Even though I was training to be a nurse, try as I might, I could not be as tolerant as I would have wished. I was still only nineteen years old, and it showed.

By the end of the week, the constant interruptions had become intensely irritating, and I became more energetic in my complaints. This was the signal that I was ready to graduate to the open ward. It was also the beginning of the long, hard process of getting well and dealing with my new body. I was visited by an enterostomal therapist (ET), a nurse with specialized training who teaches patients and families to care for a colostomy, or any kind of ostomy. She came into my room, and said: "Tell me where it is." I looked at her quizzically. "Where what is?" I asked. "My ileostomy," she replied. This ET also had an ileostomy! My eyes searched her abdomen but I couldn't see where she was hiding it. She began describing her own struggle to accept the stoma. I quickly felt comforted: here was a married woman with two children doing a real job and she had an ileostomy. She was even able to wear snug-fitting clothes. As she talked, I kept searching her waist to find it. That day, with her help, I began to confront my ileostomy—physically and emotionally.

Ostomy care and nutrition were two key concerns in my recovery. I'd been fed intravenously for four weeks, waiting for the time my bowels would accept food. Finally, the big day arrived and the doctors decided I should be given clear fluids, a meal tray appeared three times a day. The trays were laden with Jell-O (which comes in an array of colors but always tastes the same), ginger ale, apple juice, and the infamous Choice Chicken Broth, which tastes like last week's dishwater from the local fried chicken joint.

After a few days, the doctors were convinced that clear fluids would journey from one end of my gastrointestinal tract to the other. They decreed that I was ready for some real food. My first meal was lunch and, after not eating for weeks, I was very excited. In anticipation, I watched my mother lift the steamy, silver-plate dish cover. Beneath sat a sad little piece of mystery meat, accompanied by withered vegetables and parslied potatoes. My mother looked at me and, suddenly, everything came apart. I began to cry. All the pain, suffering and indignity of the hospitalization and the ileostomy came crashing down on what was left of a very frail, emotional foundation. We sat for a long time and she listened intently as my fears and frustrations poured out.

What if I couldn't go back to school? What if people found out about my ileostomy? What if I got sick again? What if I needed another operation? What if Jack rejected me?

For each fear raised, there was another close behind it. The afternoon shadows got longer, the cold meal was finally whisked away, untouched and forgotten.

The technical aspects of ostomy care were easy for me because of my training as a nurse. The ET would come into my room and change the clear plastic bag that was over my stoma. There were many steps but, as I watched her run through them, I picked up the routine. After four days, she informed me that I would start changing my own bag the next day. I worried about remembering all the steps. The following morning she arrived to help me do the task. As she peeled back the bag and I started to wash the skin around this "rosebud," I started to cry. For the first time, the stoma was real for me. I went through the steps: applying a toothpaste-like skin barrier around the stoma so any intestinal contents, which are full of skin-irritating enzymes, wouldn't cause any problems; then placing the bag over the stoma and making sure that the opening was perfectly centered. The exercise seemed reasonably easy but doing it left me emotionally exhausted. Each day, I got better at the technique, but I still couldn't look at my body and accept that it was mine.

Hospital food became an issue, as did my continuing weight loss. I didn't like the food choices and became extremely picky. Although I never felt hungry, I was given strict orders to eat. When I was first admitted to the hospital, I had weighed 112 pounds. I was down to 86 pounds, and falling, and was told I couldn't go home until I weighed 88 pounds. Although gaining two pounds sounds easy enough, to me it seemed as difficult as gaining twenty. My parents called me before each visit and insisted that I let them bring cinnamon buns smeared with butter, homemade soups, pastries from favorite downtown restaurants—anything that would trigger my appetite. They gave me bites of all my requested goodies each hour. Ounce by ounce, the weight returned.

During this time, one of my greatest fears was that anyone outside my circle of family and intimate friends would find out about my ileostomy. Each time I told a chosen friend or family member, I found myself grieving and crying all over again, recalling the first time I realized that this new body was mine forever. Usually we cried together. And then they'd leave, grateful that the calamity had struck someone else. Those I told, I swore to secrecy. I eventually posted a sign on my door asking other visitors to check at the front desk before they came to my room.

A couple of days after the sign went up, my surgeon walked into the room and announced that he was going to give me his "kick in the ass" talk. He told me that I had to stop hiding behind signs on doors and start dealing with my new body. He warned me about prolonging my re-entry into the real world and that I would have to stop hiding behind my illness. I remember feeling very angry and hurt, unsure that I was ready to move on. A few days later, I was discharged. And all my doubts went home with me.

FIVE

Going Home

The idea of going home was so wonderful that I could barely wait to check out. By the time we reached the car with all my things, I was exhausted. Six weeks had gone by since that eventful day in the emergency room. I had suffered devastating losses. It would be years before I discovered how much I'd also gained.

Mom drove slowly so I could reacquaint myself with familiar streets. Everything seemed either bigger or smaller than it had before. I was like a child returning home from a trip: the familiar had become strange, and had to be rediscovered. We chatted as we drove. I asked about the family and Mom reported on who was doing what with whom. This gossip was typical of our conversation. I marveled that life could suddenly seem so normal. After waiting and wishing so often to be going home, I was now simply going home.

When we arrived twenty minutes later, I curled up on the couch and slept for four hours. Friends and family called all day to assure themselves that I was all right and to book visiting time while my mother tried to protect me from too much company and excitement.

During one of these visits, a close friend revealed a rumor was circulating that I had stomach cancer and was dying. I was angry at myself for fostering the air of secrecy that seeded this idea. It was evident that I needed to provide honest, straightforward information to close friends.

This was the beginning of my lifelong struggle to cope with my disease. In spite of the people around me, I know I travel this journey alone. I spend my life confronting daily obstacles. I never like my illness—I usually hate it—but I have learned how to accept that hate and go on. I would feel cheated if I let it rob me of the happiness my parents gave me in giving me life.

SIX

Getting Help

You and Your Doctors

The first step toward getting help is accepting that you
have a problem. The fact that you are reading this
book means that you have decided to learn more about
coping with your illness. If you want to know how to
cope, you must have decided that you have an illness
to cope with. Good for you—you're on your way.

At what point do we decide that we need help? For
some of us, it's before we are diagnosed. For others, it
may be many years after a diagnosis is made. Whenever
it happens, it takes tremendous courage to finally reach
out, beyond our personal suffering, and seek help.

The first step may be calling that gastroenterologist's
office number, scribbled on a crumpled piece of paper
and buried in your wallet. Or it may be an informal discussion with your regular doctor, a close friend or a family
member, when those deep, disturbing fears bubble to the
surface. In almost every case, we reach out for help when
our secret symptoms begin taking over or altering our
lives so dramatically that we can no longer carry on.

The response of the first person we pour out our fears is critical in determining what we do next. If, after taking the big step, that person is negative or patronizing, we tend to pull back. Feeling vulnerable and weak, we give ourselves another reason not to pursue this any further. Most of us look for reasons to affirm what we want to believe, rather than accepting what is really happening. Like the woman with a lump in her breast, fearing what the doctor might find, we become paralyzed by the conflict between the desire to know the truth and the desire to run away from it.

People with chronic illnesses that are difficult to diagnose and treat often get caught in this trap. Medical personnel find these people less than gratifying to treat, and lose interest very quickly. If symptoms are vague and test results inconclusive, the illness may be labeled as psychosomatic or stress-related. Although some symptoms of chronic disease are clearly associated with times of stress, it is difficult to tell whether stress causes the symptoms or the symptoms cause the stress.

Regardless of the negative reactions you encounter during your career with chronic illness, don't despair. **Stand firm when you know how you feel.** Remember that you are unique and important. No one but you can feel what you are feeling. You are the only one who can relate this information accurately.

Doctors see people like you every day, as do nurses, secretaries, medical technicians and receptionists. Constant contact with sick people dulls their sensitivity to a patient's fears and interferes with their ability to treat you as the unique individual that you are. Some of them would like to take a strong personal interest in every aspect of your care, but time constraints and huge numbers of patients rarely allow that to happen. This reality leads me to a crucial piece of advice: **Be your own advocate.** Look out for yourself and speak up for yourself to make sure you are getting the best treatment available. (This does not mean that you should be pushy, negative or belligerent; those attitudes just make people want to avoid you.) You must learn how to pursue help so you don't get lost in the shuffle of a busy hospital or a crowded medical practice.

It's important to carefully **select a doctor** with whom you work well. Because of the nature of chronic illness, you will inevitably develop a long-term relationship with your doctor. Develop a friendly relationship with the receptionist, too. Ensure that the receptionist knows your name and who you are. Be courteous and ask how she is. Many busy doctors instruct their receptionists to be intimidating over the phone in order to weed out the people who do not require immediate assistance. Do not allow this trick of the trade to prevent you from seeing your doctor if you need to. Having the receptionist as your ally is one of the smartest moves you can make.

When you have tests done, find out who will be interpreting them, and when you should expect to hear the results. If you haven't heard by the time the doctor said you should, call the office to ensure that the results were received. Inquire if the doctor has seen them. In large centers, test results and other things may get lost, misplaced or put to one side. Always be polite and patient, but firm. When you do get the results, make sure you understand what they mean, even if you need the explanation repeated over and over. When you take an active interest in your results, you are apt to feel more in control.

You will be better able to understand your physician's plan, and, sensing your interest, your doctor will respond more positively to you.

We are difficult patients for our doctors. They feel the same frustration that we feel. Doctors feel most gratified by **curing** their patients. The Hippocratic oath, which all doctors must take, charges them to arrive at a cure or, if that isn't possible, to ease the suffering. Chronic illness thwarts both these goals and results in terrible frustration for doctor and patient alike. Imagine trying hard to achieve something and failing every time, no matter how hard you tried. Imagine watching someone you care for suffer, the hope and trust in their eyes turning to bitter disappointment with each new failure. It is important, from time to time, to put ourselves in our doctors' shoes, and see the situation from their perspective. This type of comprehension and sharing will create an environment within which you and your doctor can work best. The two of you are a team doing battle with this illness. If you work together, you may win more than you lose; if you don't, you are doomed before you start.

Sometimes a rift develops between you which breaks the team apart. I had a surgeon who believed that I would be better off without my remaining diseased bowel. Having had my share of operations, I loathed the prospect of another one. The general anesthetic, the dreaded third-day post-op blues and the long recuperation all haunted me. The operation that he proposed would leave me with a permanent ileostomy and no hope of reversal in the future. Each time I was admitted to the hospital with a flare-up, and was nursed back to health with conservative, nonsurgical treatment, he would visit me. Standing at the foot of my bed, he would express his fears about the drugs I was on, calling them poisons. He was genuinely concerned for my welfare, and truly believed that what he recommended was the best treatment for me. The result, however, was that these interactions made me angry and ambivalent. They left me feeling very afraid, alone and confused in my fight. I felt pressure to comply with what he thought was right, but I simply wasn't ready for the surgery yet.

The relationship with my gastroenterologist matured in a very different fashion. I learned to put up with the hours spent in his waiting room because, once inside his office, I was allowed as much time as I needed. He spent time with me, catching up on how I was doing and inquiring about the changes in my life, both physical and emotional. My greatest support came from the endless supply of anecdotes about someone just like me who had responded well to a given treatment and was still doing fine. New drug regimens were accompanied by information designed to reduce my fear of side effects. Liquid nutritional supplements were tasted and often tossed, with no guilt or admonishments.

The time that I was most acutely aware of his support was during a prolonged admission to hospital for bed rest and intravenous nutrition. One afternoon, while I was crying and contemplating suicide with the thought of losing the rest of my large bowel, he quietly entered the room. I was staring out the window at the city skyline, my back to the door. Pulling up a chair so that his face was in line with mine, he outlined clearly and concisely how he planned to add a new drug to my treatment that he was sure would work. His certainty was infectious.

He outlined my responsibilities, step by step, bringing me into the therapeutic plan as a co-conspirator. In allowing me to be a part of my own destiny, he encouraged me to channel my energy away from despair and towards recovery. Whether or not his optimism was justified, and whether or not the change in plan was really for the better, he made me an integral part of the team. The drug he really offered me that afternoon was hope.

People Around You

At times during the course of a chronic illness, our greatest handicap becomes our helplessness. When our needs exceed our own capabilities and those of our partners and our doctors, we may need to turn to friends and family to keep order in our lives.

It is important to distinguish the real offers of help from the superficial ones. People trying to appear thoughtful will offer their help. Beware of depending on people who utter the phrase, **"If there is anything I can do, please let me know,"** without any specific suggestions before or after the offer. It is too difficult to translate this offer into something useful. These would-be helpers have just relieved themselves of the guilt they feel for enjoying the luxury of good health. They have offered their healthy selves for your personal use. The onus is on you to suggest what they should do to help you. Of course, you feel guilty for demanding something specific, especially if it may take time or effort.

When people are serious about helping you, they will immediately suggest something concrete like babysitting, cooking or taking on one of your responsibilities at work. It's far easier to deal with specific suggestions than with open-ended ones. Remember that you really do need help. Accept and fine-tune all offers. Help the people who want to help you by telling them exactly what you need. Learn to work with others. Show your appreciation by sending flowers, candy or other expressions of thanks. These gestures go a long way to keep up your end of the relationship.

Our needs range from the very basic to the extremely complex. The following two lists contain key examples. The first one outlines tasks you may need help with during hospitalization. The second list describes daily needs: basic long-term requirements that will allow you adequate rest, so that you can achieve and maintain the firmest possible hold on health. These are the kind of specific activities that people can take on to help you out.

Hospitalization Needs

Arranging food for your family at home
Babysitting for your children
Getting your children to and from school and other activities
Getting your children to and from the hospital to see you
Laundering your family's clothing
Cleaning your home
Discharging your job-related responsibilities
Bringing articles from home to the hospital (clean clothes, personal items, reading material)

Bringing in special foods

Providing you with an ear, bringing news from the outside (especially good gossip), providing laughter

Sharing hobbies such as word puzzles, knitting, painting or board games, video games, video movies, a laptop computer

Visiting you in the hospital and keeping abreast of your medical progress

Providing financial help when needed

Daily Needs

Babysitting your children while you are resting

Answering the phone while you are resting

Visiting and listening

Bringing news from the outside world

Entertaining and sharing enjoyable activities

Cooking meals

Shopping

Keeping your home clean

Laundry

Driving you to and from medical appointments

Helping get your children to their activities and school

Asking for help is one of the most difficult ongoing tasks you will have. If you were a person who found it difficult to ask for help before you were ill, your feelings are not likely to change. What *will* change is how badly you need the help. You won't be able to survive without it. Not being in the position now or in the foreseeable future to repay a kindness can also provoke intense feelings of guilt.

Guilt can be very destructive to any relationship: no matter what you do, it colors all interactions. You never feel finished. You are always in the process of justifying yourself and repaying others. It's not your fault that you are chronically ill and need help. Seek out the kind of help that provokes the least amount of guilt. Rather than ask your old stand-bys for yet another favor, pay a neighbor's son or daughter to help you cut the lawn, shop for groceries or babysit your kids at a local playground. Paying a small fee for these kinds of services often minimizes the long-term toll on your guilt meter, and avoids straining important friendships. You may want to save the favors from friends for emergency situations.

I wish I knew a way around the helplessness that is created by chronic illness. I wish I could wave a magic wand and we would all enjoy good health and the ability to care for ourselves and our dependants. Unfortunately, these wishes are simply fantasies.

I had a terrible flare-up when my daughter was seventeen months old. Perhaps it was because I became so sick, or perhaps it was because a child was now in the picture, but it was the first time I felt that I could not take care of my life if I was hospitalized. I hung on to this idea day by day as my illness intensified. I started to examine how I was feeling every hour. I had conversations in my head. "I think I feel a little better now," said the optimistic, unrealistic me. And, "Maybe I'll get better without needing to be admitted to that awful place."

The next few hours would be filled with pain, nausea and the overwhelming need to lie down. My pessimistic, realistic side would say, "See, the doctor's right. You can't do it without help." Each day, the dialogue continued.

One afternoon, in the playground, I no longer felt safe caring for Jessica. I felt faint and all I wanted to do was collapse. She kept pulling on my clothes to get me to play with her. It was then I finally realized that I needed help.

Jessica went to my mother's, and I went to the hospital. Despite my anxiety, I was so sick and exhausted I slept for the entire first week. When I was discharged five weeks later, I was ready to take on some of my old responsibilities again, I felt that I had gotten over a tremendous hurdle. It was a rough time for everyone, but it worked out well because we had a defined goal. My goal was to get well enough to resume my life as quickly and as normally as possible. Asking for help from friends and family was the easiest, most reliable way to achieve that goal.

When you ignore the signals your illness gives you and push yourself beyond the limit, you hurt yourself and those who depend on you. Once you learn how to care for yourself, you'll be better able to care for those around you. It is very difficult to accept help from others no matter how much you need them. Realize that the love you share with your friends and family goes beyond the boundaries of only good times. These people love you for the person you are, even with your illness. It is your job to trust their love and to accept their help, free of guilt and free of chains.

SEVEN

Family and Friends

Most of us find it difficult to discuss our disease with anyone but our family and close friends. These are the people with whom we feel comfortable expressing our innermost feelings. When I am ill, I talk to my husband. It is very important to find someone who truly listens to you.

Interestingly enough, the biggest problem arises when I am feeling well and trying to deny that my disease exists. When I ignore it, I expect others to do the same. I sometimes don't give the people around me the chance to switch gears from their role as listener to their role as accomplice in denial. The simplest question from my mother such as "How are you feeling?" can bring out the absolute worst in me, if I am not in the mood to discuss how I am feeling. Unreasonably, I wish she could just know which days I don't want to talk about *it*.

I look for ulterior motives behind simple questions. For instance, when one of my brothers commented on how healthy I looked, I assumed it was because my face was puffy from prednisone. I hated the side effect from that medication. It always made me feel so distorted and so unlike myself. My first reaction was to interpret his comment as an insult rather than a compliment, and get upset. When I am feeling well, I don't want people commenting on my health—I want people to treat me like I am not ill.

This, of course, isn't fair. With chronic illness, it's too easy to become self-absorbed: we owe it to our loved ones and close friends to recognize that they have concerns for our well-being. They experience the illness with us, suffering every step of the way. How they respond and how much they are able to give depends on many things.

We often get angry and disappointed when close friends find it difficult to help when we need them. We forget that they need direction. We are so accustomed to being cared for that we don't care for the people who take care of us. By giving back some of the same consideration and understanding that we so desperately need, we give them something invaluable.

It is more fun to be with people who provide some form of entertainment or psychological stimulation. Illness makes people plaintive, wrapped up—as they are—in their bodily functions and needs. When we feel unwell, we can't do the things we normally do or concentrate on anything outside ourselves. The activities that we shared with others are no longer common ground. A tennis game or a simple walk in the park may be unthinkable.

We feel that we are boring and become angry towards others for not understanding the sacrifices required of us because we are sick. Chronic illness can force us to give up a beloved job, stop us from having children, or simply prevent us from being able to get around because of the pain. When help is offered we may be too angry to accept it.

When we talk about how we feel, our audience starts to dwindle. We can become so focused that all we talk about is the illness. Old friends often find it difficult to be with us.

I remember attending a party. I had been feeling moderately ill for about six months. As people asked, "How are you?" I responded with the usual "not bad." That evening, though, I decided to dispense with the inane civility and say how I was really feeling. My test elicited a variety of responses. One friend asked, "So, how are ya?" to which I replied, "Awful, just awful. I'm really tired of being in the hospital some of the time and in the bathroom the rest of the time. It doesn't leave time for very much else." My friend reacted with uncomfortable silence and, at the earliest possible moment, found an excuse to leave my corner of the room. Perhaps it was mean of me to put her on the spot, but I knew she didn't want to deal with someone else's problems. I'm sure she felt trapped and helpless, not knowing what to say.

Some friends were very good listeners at first, but ultimately lapsed into avoidance of either the topic, me, or both. The only people I felt confident in sharing how I was truly feeling was my parents, my husband and a few close friends.

After a period of time, we all get depressed listening to ourselves talk about how awful we feel. When we really listen to ourselves, we hear about this unfortunate person, and we think, "Hey, who is that they're talking about? Poor thing. What a life." Then a sinking feeling comes over us as we remember that we are describing ourselves.

It is not hard to imagine how tedious it can get for others to continually listen to the same old story.

The feelings of guilt experienced by you and your supporters are inevitable. You are the person in need. The more ill you are, and the longer it drags on, the greater your needs become. Over time, even your best friend's patience sometimes runs out.

People with chronic illness share a comradery that is much like belonging to a club. This, however, is a club for which you did not seek membership: you were conscripted. Inside this club, everyone understands. The long explanations that outsiders require never seem to be needed. Like old friends, we share the same joy, pain and history. We each have our own stories, with individual settings and different casts of characters, but the plot keeps repeating itself over and over again. We each experience our illness alone, but the experiences bind us together. The key to finding help is finding each other.

EIGHT

Losing Control

One summer afternoon, as I was sitting in the back-yard, poring over an application for graduate school, my mom came to visit.

"How are you?" she asked, craning her neck so she could see what I was doing. I was feeling constant pain from active anal disease, and I decided that I wasn't in the mood to share that information with her.

"Not bad," I answered.

The conversation turned to the application I was filling out—she couldn't resist.

"Do you think that graduate school is such a good idea right now?" she said. "After all, you've been so sick the past six months. You really don't need any more pressure."

I usually responded defensively to this kind of remark from her, but this time I didn't. I stopped for a minute and tried to review exactly what I was doing. I had been hospitalized for one week out of every month for the past six months. I had had two examinations under anesthetic and my anal disease was producing so much pain and discomfort that I had difficulty sitting down. I was also six weeks pregnant and Jack and I were considering moving. For most people, this would have been more than enough stress. So why was I about to take on even more? Was I crazy?

The real issue here was control. In hindsight, I see now that I was feeling a lack of control in the direction my life was moving.

People need to feel some measure of control over their lives and destinies. When it is taken away, they feel very insecure. Crohn's disease had controlled my life decisions for so long I felt the need to fight back. Applying to graduate school, getting pregnant and moving were all ways of challenging my limitations, proving my self-worth. If I could change direction, then I could take over as captain of my destiny.

The more I look back at the basic issues surrounding gaining and losing control with chronic illness, the more I believe it to be the most debilitating aspect of the sufferer's life. This is and will continue to be a recurring theme in our lives.

When I feel ill, any changes in my life have to be made and suggested by *me*. If my mother sees that I am tired and offers to babysit for my children for a couple of hours, I become annoyed. If, on the other hand, *I* decide I need a break and call on my mom to help, it feels better. I do the asking; I am in control. If that sounds like adolescence revisited, remember, illness makes us regress. Explain this to the people who love and support you; it will help them feel less hurt or rejected.

The times that are hardest for me are when I am incapacitated at home or in the hospital and other people must take over my responsibilities. This is difficult to cope with, especially if, like me, you lean towards perfectionism and like everything "just so."

When Jack came down to the hospital with Jessica one morning to visit me, she came bouncing into the room all smiles and hugs. All I could see after her initial hello was that she didn't have pretty clips in her hair and her socks and shoes didn't match. I was upset at Jack and he couldn't understand my frustration. Let's face it, the clips and shoes were not the real issue. What I couldn't bear then, and cannot stand to this day, is the feeling of being replaced in my role as mother. I felt dispensable.

Over the years, I have learned to be more open about the things that really bother me so that I can try to control them and leave the rest to others. Jessica's hair is a good example. No one else can ever seem to do it "just right." I don't try to hide the fact that relatively minor issues take on greater importance when I'm sick. I now realize that constant hospitalization deprives me of so much control that any aggressiveness over additional losses (no matter how trivial) is natural. But, as well, I've learned to let some things go and not take issue with every situation. Jack and I now joke about the hair clips, especially since Jessica is old enough to wear her hair the way she wants to.

Over the years, I have learned to be more open about the things that really bother me, so that I can try to control them and leave the rest to others. Jessica's hair is a good example. No one else can ever seem to do it "right." I don't try to hide my feelings about this, or other relatively minor issues that somehow take on greater importance when I am sick. I try to be open and honest. Jack and I joke about it now, especially since she is old enough to wear it the way *she* wants to. I have learned to let some things go and not take issue with every situation. When you are hospitalized, so many of your rights, so much of your individuality and sense of control are removed that you may become aggressive over any additional losses, no matter how trivial.

The dependency that accompanies chronic illness places you in the perpetual role of a child. It's hard to grow up when you are constantly dependant. Your parents or partner may, through no fault of their own, be placed in the role of tending to your needs as if you were still a small child.

One six month stretch, I was perpetually ill and constantly in and out of the hospital. I had a dilemma. Although I was a parent myself, I was being mothered by my mother and fathered by my father. I felt like a young child. I wanted them to take over. I felt so ill I didn't want to make the decisions, and I wanted my parents to make them for me.

Once I started to feel better, I rejected my mother's mothering. I would go out of my way to pull silly stunts and show her I didn't need her help. One afternoon, when I was in the hospital, she called to say she would come by and help me wash my hair. I could not get out of bed easily, had an intravenous in my arm, and had recently had abdominal surgery. By the time she arrived, I was sitting on my bed with my hair washed and blown dry and trying very hard to conceal my cold sweat.

"I thought you wanted me to help you with your hair," she said in a hurt tone.

"It's all right. I managed by myself," I proudly replied.

It's important to talk about these role changes and control issues. Tell your partner, parents and close friends how difficult it is to lose control—and thank them for their help when you need it, and tell them no thanks when you feel ready to resume your independence.

Loss of control as a result of illness is a well-documented phenomenon in the health-care field. It affects people of all ages and stages of life. Having a chronic illness can make you feel as if your life is on a hijacked plane. Each one perceives it differently, but losing control of one's life is at the top of the heap of complaints about chronic illness. Communication is the key to your survival. Nothing you do can change the fact that you will lose control many times in your life. Learn to be open, talk about your feelings; you will achieve the strength to carry on until you can get behind the wheel again.

NINE

The Pain Drain

Pain

Both emotional and physical, pain is an integral part of all chronic illness. The emotional pain is intertwined with the physical. One incites the other, and both can leave you feeling helpless and hopeless. The pain can be so profound at times it causes intense grief and a desire to give in and give up.

Pain is part of the loneliness of chronic illness. As you look around you in a crowded room, on the bus or walking down the street, you wonder if people know what it feels like to spend each day struggling to keep your head above water.

After I had had Crohn's disease for eight years, I discovered the essence to coping with incapacitating chronic pain. Whatever daily pain I'd experienced before, I was able to control with over-the-counter headache-type medication. I had no idea what real chronic pain was all about. During that summer, eight years ago, I learned.

I developed severe anal Crohn's disease. No matter what I did to rid myself of the pain, it stayed with me.

When I went to bed each night, it was there, hanging on the edge of my consciousness, thwarting my attempts to sleep. When I woke, its ugly face was there to greet me. My energy level became increasingly poor. I knew that energy loss was a symptom of my disease flaring up. After a while I realized that all my available energy was pouring into the bottomless pit of pain control.

I was lying in bed one night, trying to fall asleep, when it suddenly dawned on me. I had been fighting a guerrilla war with this pain for six months, and it was clearly winning. I was short-tempered with my husband, my little girl, even with strangers in the street. Everything in my life seemed to be melting into one big chore. The joy lacking from my days was not rejuvenated as I tossed and turned each night waiting for the sandman, who seemed to have forgotten where I lived.

Chronic pain depletes a person's physical and emotional strength. It interferes with the ability to cope with life's everyday events. If you see through a shroud of pain, it is soon difficult to see anything clearly. Each of us begins our day with available energy. Most healthy people do not use the entire allotment. Disappointments, work deadlines, sickness, family crises and other stresses deplete the coffers of even the healthiest person. If you have to spend a third, or more, of your energy strictly coping with pain, you become exhausted. There is no gratification in it. It is like an albatross hanging around your neck, dragging you down.

Unfortunately, there may not be an easy solution. It may be the result of an active disease process. The overwhelming experience of being chronically ill may cause you excruciating emotional pain.

There are many available methods of pain control. Some people simply take stronger medication. Although this is a solution that may control or dull the pain, the side effects and the potential for addiction may have serious implications for your life. The trade-off is usually not worth it. Codeine taken in small doses is used frequently in Canada because it is readily available without a prescription. This medication can cause drowsiness and poor performance when fine motor tasks, or other situations requiring strict attention, are attempted. Narcotics such as these can also be very addictive. What starts off as an innocent attempt to control pain may result in a new, separate but equally incapacitating problem. The medications can mask larger problems and dupe the user into forgetting that the underlying illness expresses itself by causing pain. Masking it with increasing doses may cause important warning signs to be ignored. On the other hand, if used in small, reasonable doses, narcotics can be a good solution by providing the freedom necessary to carry on with the activities of daily life.

There are other methods of dealing with the pain besides drugs. Hypnosis is used for many diverse conditions in the 1990s. This is a sleeplike condition, psychically induced, during which a person loses consciousness but is able, within certain limitations, to respond to the suggestions of the hypnotist. Hypnotic suggestion to the unconscious may allow the patient to ignore painful sensations. Acupuncture, which has been practiced in Asian cultures for thousands of years, is another alternative to traditional Western medicine. Transcendental meditation and creative visualization, two other approaches, can help the person achieve complete relaxation by focusing mental energy. (Relaxation directly affects pain perception, and provides the body with a boost of energy.) The French obstetrician Dr. Lamaze, who developed techniques for pain control during labor, was the first to popularize the concept of focused energy and relaxation. Women learn to breathe rhythmically, call the pain "contractions" and stimulate alternate nerve pathways by rubbing their abdomen (effleurage). Finally, pain clinics can be very useful. These clinics teach people to change their lifestyle and focus on healthy, active living. Clinics like these also provide a forum for mutual support and encouragement.

I don't know of any sure-fire methods to take away your pain. I certainly wish that I did. Pain will get worse or subside according to the ebb and flow of your illness. When you have a chronic illness you learn to accept a lot of things in your life you don't like. Pain, unfortunately, is one of them. The most constructive solution I can offer is to re-evaluate your goals and expectations during the days, weeks or months that the pain is truly incapacitating. Recognize and respect your pain. If you try to carry on as if nothing unusual is happening, it will ultimately bring you down.

Practical Suggestions for Living with Pain

What follows are some specific ground rules which I have found helpful in accomplishing my tasks and which leave me less tired at the end of a working day. The basic principle is to take as much pressure off yourself as possible while still fulfilling your responsibilities.

1) Look at your responsibilities and list them. From the list, circle those things that are imperative for the household, office or store to continue functioning.

2) Plan things out carefully from a sitting position, comfortably in a quiet atmosphere. Give yourself at least ten minutes to do this, so that you can organize your plan clearly. A good time to do this may be after the children are in bed and the telephone has stopped ringing for the night. I find that I can relax and think best in a shower or bath. After I have gone through this exercise in my mind it is a piece of cake to put down on paper.

3) Identify things that someone else can assist you with, or can be accomplished more easily by a different method. For example, if you can have your groceries delivered rather than having to do the shopping, go for it. If you can hire someone to shovel the driveway or cut the grass, hire them. This can be costly, but it is all part of re-adjusting the expectations you have of yourself, and making them more realistic.

4) Pace yourself, and try not to pack too much into each day. Carefully plan out an errand route so you don't have to backtrack.

5) Each day should contain protected time for personal grooming. If you are in pain and think that you look worse than you feel, your attitude will reflect it. Spending a little extra time on yourself may give you an emotional boost.

6) Plan rest periods as an important part of your day. Sacrifice some other chore: you will be the big loser if you don't get enough rest. Exhaustion will make you vulnerable, and the pain can be paralyzing.

Children

For those of you with children to care for, here are other concrete suggestions to help you meet your responsibilities and conserve energy.

1) Get the chldren up and dressed. Teach your children to use an alarm clock, and praise them for their independence. Put out clothing the night before so there are no arguments in the morning. Purchase clothing that requires a minimal amount of help from you (i.e. velcro and zippers rather than laces and buttons). Praise them again for their independence.
2) Put Breakfast on the table. Plan nutritious, easy meals that the children like and can prepare.
3) Get children to school. Sometimes a neighbor's older child can walk your child to school. It's best to reward the helping child with a nominal fee. School principals and classroom teachers can help you put together this kind of arrangement. Or, does your child's school have a transportation program that you can take advantage of? You may just need help with the mornings. If you are in a carpool, be up front with carpool members, and try to choose a schedule that suits you best so you won't have to cancel at the last minute. Your child will feel disappointed if you cannot drive when you said you would.
4) Get children to playgroup. Choose playgroup programs that are in your neighborhood or not too far away. If necessary, try to arrange a carpool. Evaluate cooperative programs so that you know how much

responsibility you are expected to take. Generally it is easier if you choose a program that doesn't require your participation. You don't need the additional stress.

5) Shopping. Whenever possible, buy your groceries in bulk. This strategy will also cover the times you may be hospitalized unexpectedly. With twenty-four-hour shopping available in some communities, your partner may be able to help by doing the main weekly shopping.

6) Cooking. When you cook a meal, make enough for two meals and freeze the rest. It will be available on the days when you feel too ill to cook and don't want your family to have another take-out meal. If friends or family offer to make a meal for you and your family, or offer to take you out, take them up on it.

7) Housekeeping. Hire someone to do the heavy housework, and reward conscientious clean-up behavior in the household. Housecleaning often suffers the most because of its low priority, yet ongoing messiness may have its own emotional stresses.

8) Post office, banking. Can usually be done by your partner, or, a friend who is going to run those errands anyway.

9) Drycleaners. Try to engage the pick-up drop-off service. Car pool children to after-school activities. Be up-front with carpool members and try to choose a schedule in which you can be most reliable. Your child will feel disappointed if you can not drive when you said you would. There is status involved in their mommy or daddy being the driver.

10) Easy activities with the children. Pain days are not the time to embark on full day outings to the zoo.

Bring out that rainy day cache of toys and watch from a lying down or relaxed position. Video movies may be the ticket on some days. Quiet indoor activity may not hold out for the entire playtime. Purchase outdoor equipment so that you can watch the children from the penned in safety of your own backyard. If you don't have a backyard find a small neighbourhood playground (preferably with bathroom facilities). Don't underestimate the amount of energy needed just to go out the door.

11)Talk to your spouse. Be honest about the amount of help you need. Remember to express your appreciation. Spend some quiet time together on a regular basis.

Personal Needs

1) Daily shower, make-up, hair. Some people find that the best time for taking their shower and doing their make-up and hair is before the kids get up. If you have early-risers this may be impossible. Try to find time during their nap or their favorite TV show.

2) Nutrition. Don't skip meals. You need the well-being that comes from good nutrition. Feed yourself the way you want your children to eat.

3) Exercise. Staying in good physical shape gives you a positive feeling about yourself, and decreases your level of stress. But be careful not to overdo it. Pace yourself. If you belong to a club, studio or YMCA, advise them that you may be ill for periods of time and ask if your membership could have a flexible time limit. If possible, buy individual classes rather than a series. Most clubs will be understanding.

4) Give yourself time to think quietly. You need some
   time for psychological rejuvenation. Reading a good
   novel or the newspaper, practicing meditation or listening to music all fall into this category. Sometimes
   my best source of pain relief is a good hot bath, some
   classical music and a trashy novel.

Re-evaluate your day when you feel that the pain and
your daily responsibilities are overwhelming you. Try to
reorganize your activities so that you can maximize your
energy conservation and minimize your stress. If you deplete your energy resources you won't be able to function
in a way that expresses who you are and want to be.
This causes more emotional and physical pain, and further
depletes your energy resources. It is a vicious cycle that
must be broken. When faced with adversity, we often tend
to push ourselves harder, but fighting the pain doesn't
make it go away. By learning to live with the daily menu
it serves up each day, you learn to live in harmony with
pain.

TEN

I Hate Taking Medications

As I rifled through my personal and make-up cases and picked up my purse to start searching through it, I shouted down the stairs to Jack: "Have you seen my pills anywhere?" We were away for the weekend and it was at least a thirty-minute drive to a pharmacy that *might* stock the medications I needed.

I can no longer recall the number of times this, and similar scenes, has taken place. Ever since I started taking pills to help control my disease, they have been an issue. The problems range from simply forgetting to take them, to the side effects and the game-playing by consciously omitting them from my daily routine. There are many drug therapies, in many different combinations, which make up the Crohn's disease patient's therapeutic regime. At the time of my initial diagnosis, I received corticosteroids intravenously to reduce the inflammation in my very inflamed bowels. After my first surgery, the oral form of the drug—prednisone—was used to combat the disease in my remaining bowel. As soon as I was well enough to travel, Jack and I took a three-week trip to the East

Coast of Canada. Taking large doses of prednisone, I felt well and had a wonderful time. I even found the ileostomy manageable. I looked at myself everyday in the mirror but didn't see my slowly expanding cheeks. All I saw was a healthy glow. The Prince Edward Island sun contributed to a wonderful tan and the hospital pallor became exorcised from my skin. Jack saw me everyday and didn't notice that my face had changed, nor did the people we met along our journey.

We arrived home in time to go to one of my oldest and dearest friend's wedding. I could not have been prepared for the reaction of my friends. Most of them passed me by as if I was invisible. I started to become concerned. What was wrong? Why wouldn't anyone talk to me? I went over to an old friend. "Hi, Mark. How are you?" I said. He must have recognized my voice. "God, Ferne," he said, "what happened to your face?" My heart started to pound. Suddenly, I realized why everyone was ignoring me. My face had become so distorted that no one even recognized me. Once people realized who I was, they averted their eyes as they asked me how I was. I was so embarrassed. All I wanted to do was go home. At the earliest moment, I bid my thanks and farewells and went home to cry myself to sleep.

This distortion of my features was a condition I became accustomed to for about one full year. During that time, I heard it all. My brother-in-law thought I looked like a "chipmunk storing nuts for the winter." But my favorite one was from a fellow student in Criminology 101. "Hi Ferne," he said. "Gee, I didn't realize that you had your wisdom teeth out." By that time, I was so tired of the remarks that I turned abruptly and looked him straight in the eye. "I didn't," I said, and turned on my heel and walked away. It was no one's fault, but the emotional pain of taking the pill was becoming so severe that I started playing games with them.

At first, it was truly forgetfulness. I would forget to take my pills in the morning, have none in my purse, and be out all day at school and clinic. Then it would be the end of the day, if I still felt fine I would simply skip them for that day. The next day I would take them, but the day after I wouldn't. I would keep a close eye on my symptoms and found myself, on a number of occasions, choking back catch-up pills if any symptoms did arise. This game was strictly between me and my pills.

The reasons were obvious. I loved my pills because they were helping to keep my disease under control, allowing me to go to school and stay out of the hospital as a full-time boarder. The hate was directly related to the embarrassment and frustration of having to look at my cushingoid moon face. Anyway you slice it, having a distorted face that didn't feel or look like me was awful. So the medication game began, and continues—on and off—to this very day.

Soon I was to realize that the distortion was not confined to physical symptoms. Anyone who has ever been on prednisone will tell you about the emotional rollercoaster rides it gives free, without the asking. The higher doses leave you with a feeling of tremendous energy and, at times, euphoria. You don't need sleep; you are often hungry and eat non-stop, potentially causing you to gain large amounts of weight. Once the dose is tapered, the world suddenly feels like a very cruel, awful place where no one understands you. You feel like you have the flu and your blood pressure and sugar-level swings can make you feel faint. Sleep becomes something you can't get enough of: the opposite of when you are on high doses. Your appetite starts to ease off. Even if you are prepared for an emotional and physical low, this is a terrible time. Try not to make major decisions during these times of mini-crises.

Sometimes, while on prednisone, I feel completely out of control, as if I'm going insane. I don't have answers for why I feel as if I am going crazy at the time. In hindsight, I'd point my finger at prednisone as the major culprit although even the experienced drug consumer can be fooled.

There are many drug therapies used in the treatment of Crohn's disease and all chronic illnesses. Each one has its own glory and its demons. What should we do about the ambivalence we feel towards taking these drugs? In medicine and nursing, compliance is the key to successful treatment. Compliance means simply following the instructions. If we follow instructions, we have a much better chance of staying well for longer periods of time. When the doctor tells you to take three pills a day, human nature tells you that two should really work. By the time you forget one, you are down to only one a day. If you don't get any kick-back from the disease, you may soon be down to none.

Try not to be your own doctor! Your doctor can not give you his or her best when you are fooling around on the side. If you are unhappy about the drugs you are taking and want them changed, dropped or rearranged, **talk to your doctor**. If you don't, he or she may not know why you are responding so poorly to prescribed treatment, which you are not taking. It's always a problem when you disagree with your doctor about the management of your illness. If you cannot resolve this problem, it may be time to get yourself a new doctor you can work with. If you are going to play games (and we all do), remember that a fat face is still a face that is part of a body that can function. Having a thin face and drug-free body may cost you your health and your freedom. Recognize that this will be an ongoing theme, and work toward finding compromises that will satisfy both you and your doctor.

ELEVEN

Partnership and Having Children

Partnership

I always knew that I wanted to have children. After I was diagnosed with Crohn's disease, and particularly after the need for an ileostomy arose, I became sure that it would never happen. I was going to be a chronically ill woman with an ileostomy, how could I be acceptable as a sexual partner or a mother? When I was permitted only one person to accompany me to surgery for my ileostomy, I chose my boyfriend rather than my parents— I needed reassurance that I would still be accepted and desired as a sexual being. Then the next wave of doubt crashed into me: Even if I remain desirable to my partner, will I be able to conceive or carry a child in my womb after this rearrangement of my bodily functions?

As it turned out, I was fortunate on both counts. I found a partner for whom the ileostomy never mattered.

He could always see me first and ignore my limitations. I was able to conceive and carry three beautiful children. I am acutely aware, however, that many sufferers of chronic illness are not so fortunate.

A number of years ago, I had a friend who developed cancer. At the time of her diagnosis, she was seriously dating a young man. When she first got sick, he was there for her. But when the diagnosis was confirmed, and the truth hit, their relationship very quickly fell apart. He informed her that he "just couldn't handle it." She was astounded. Exactly what was it that she was asking him to handle? Some people are simply incapable of facing a crisis, particularly when it is happening to someone close to them; they find it easier to run and hide, to pretend that it's not happening. They feel their own mortality, and fear chokes their ability to give of themselves.

With chronic illness, the long haul that we face is for a lifetime, and it's better to find out at the beginning who we can count on and who we can't. Many different people will fill gaps in our lives, but most of us have one central person to help us pull it all together, someone we can depend on for day-to-day support, and during crises. By pooling our strength, we provide a more unified and stronger front against the ravages of illness.

Our partners need to learn, as we do, how to live with chronic illness, and how to experience the profound feelings that it conjures up from deep inside. **We don't want to view our lives according to all the things we can't do, can't have and can't be because of our illness. We want to be able to focus on what we can do, can have and can be.** Our shared responsibility should be honest communication, and helping each other move along the continuum of coping.

Chronic illness has an unfortunate habit of tearing people apart, isolating them from each other, because of the amount of anger, grief and despair associated with it. Each new episode may reignite old, negative feelings, established fears and arguments. The key to staying together is to open healthy lines of communication, which will strengthen with each new crisis. It is important to develop these communication patterns during times of remission, and make them a part of our daily life.

There are two basic, important rules to maximize healthy communication:

1) Whenever possible, don't poison your words with sarcasm, which is actually an indirect and destructive way of expressing anger. It is, of course, necessary and good to express anger when it is warranted. Try to formulate what you want to say, and then say it directly.

It is very difficult for the healthy person to express anger toward the ill partner. It seems wrong and generates tremendous feelings of guilt. Conversely, it is difficult for the sick partner to express anger toward the person who is holding together the pieces of their life. Only by openly discussing these feelings can we discard the anger and move forward to share other, better things. It's okay for your partner to tell you that it's terrible for him when you are sick. And it's okay for you to be angry with your partner because he won't fight harder for the nurse to give you pain medication on time. Express your frustration with the illness to each other. If you share your feelings, neither of you will have to cope with the illness in isolation.

2) Try to share your fears, hopes and dreams with each other. Keeping fears inside requires emotional energy

and breeds paralyzing anxiety. Emotional energy is valuable, and should be spent elsewhere. Once fears are out in the open, they may seem less frightening, like the monsters in a child's closet when daylight exposes them for the imposters that they are.

Having Children

Deciding

The diagnosis of a chronic illness affects many life decisions. Perhaps the most important is the decision whether or not to have children. Even under normal circumstances, this decision requires a tremendous amount of soul searching and commitment. Chronic illness, with its unpredictable and debilitating attacks, compromises our ability to look after ourselves; this challenge is difficult enough without adding the enormous responsibility of parenthood. For many of us, having a family is an integral part of our life's master plan. But it is very important to consider the support systems that we have available or will be able to cultivate so that we can better prepare for the inevitable bouts of illness.

Jack and I talked about having children when we seriously contemplated marriage. The severe inflammation that had engulfed my ovaries and tubes made it unlikely, in the doctor's opinion, that I would be able to conceive a child. We were in our early twenties and had no idea how much responsibility a child would add to our lives. Marriage—and parenthood—is always a gamble and, in our case, the cards were stacked against us from the beginning.

I am always relieved that we talked about having a family before we married. We decided that we would try to adopt children if we couldn't have our own. Many people need time to allow the shock of infertility to sink in and feel comfortable with the idea of raising an adopted child. For others, adoption is never an acceptable alternative. The options should be discussed at an early stage, before marriage, if possible, so that a mutually acceptable decision can be made.

Once we decided, I asked my gastroenterologist if he thought I was well enough to become pregnant. He cautioned me that it might take a long time to conceive, and that it might never happen. He also gave me some surprising and disturbing information. It appeared that two completely different things could happen to patients with Crohn's disease during pregnancy. Some improve and occasionally go into complete remission, while others have a severe exacerbation of the disease. "Is there any way to predict?" I asked. He shook his head. I went home feeling as if I was about to play Russian roulette.

Many chronic illnesses "run" in families. Anyone who has a genetically based disease worries about passing it on to their biological children. Would I be able to live with the guilt and pain if one of my children developed this disease? I discussed this issue on a number of occasions with my gastroenterologist. In his usual fashion, he gave me a wise, comforting answer. "My mother has diabetes in her family," he told me. "There is a good chance that I could have inherited that disease from her. Do you think my mother should have given that possibility strong consideration before she had me?" I looked at this wonderfully accomplished individual in front of me. I

realized exactly how much I would have missed him if
she had decided not to risk it.

The average person on the street has a one-in-two-
thousand chance of developing Crohn's disease. The odds
of my child developing Crohn's disease are approximately
ten times greater than the average: my children would
have a one-in-two-hundred chance. Jack and I weighed
the odds against depriving ourselves of being parents. I
was convinced that having our own children was the right
thing to do. Although there will always be the fear that
our children may get my disease, we felt that it would
be wrong to give in to fear and allow it to dictate the
course of our lives.

In today's society, many of us are achievement-oriented,
weaned on instant gratification and raised to believe that
everything in life should have a happy ending. We want
assurances that we will not have to change our master
plan. My middle-class upbringing attempted to shield me
from the disappointments of life, but I quickly learned
that it was impossible for anyone or anything to protect
me from the casualties of chronic illness.

Baby-boomers like myself are having fewer children
than previous generations did, and building higher expectations for them as if each child was our only chance
at creating a legacy. We want our children to have the
upper hand, the competitive edge, without handicaps, so
that they will come out on top. By having fewer children,
we have increased the ante.

As parents, we have a strong, protective instinct beginning with the plan to become parents and growing
by a quantum leap the moment the child is born. It's
hard to watch our children suffer. To feel responsible for

our children's suffering may feel like an insurmountable task.

Each person with a chronic illness is only too familiar with the feelings of guilt, powerlessness and fear. They are inseparable. My experience has taught me how much damage chronic illness can cause. I know how much pain it can involve. I can only guess how difficult it was for my parents to see me so ill, powerless to do anything about it. If one of my children gets the disease, I would fear the prospect of watching my child suffer. I fear that the guilt of inflicting this suffering will tear me apart.

Getting Pregnant

The decision to have a child was the first in a long list of dilemmas. Some people wouldn't contemplate the risk I was taking and would adopt a child. Would I grow to resent a child who developed my disease, through no fault of its own, and further compounded my health problems? I searched my soul for the answer.

I talked to my gynecologist about another issue: the ramifications of being pregnant while on medication. As we reviewed the drug store in my purse, I realized that (and despite everyone's reassurances) my fetus would be exposed to potentially harmful drugs, and there was little that I could do about it. If my child was deformed, would I be able to live with the guilt—and the responsibility? Was it worth the risk?

The intensity of our desire to have children ultimately made the decision for us, and we bravely plunged forward. Within two months, to our amazement, I conceived. We braced ourselves against a possible decline in my health but, on the contrary, my health improved. Soon after the pregnancy began, I was able to drop the last drug from my regime. Being drug-free for the first time in six years was almost as exciting as being pregnant.

My second pregnancy did not go so well. My disease flared up, and I was hospitalized and on intravenous nutrition for a month. I developed mysterious fevers, which could not be adequately investigated because I was pregnant. I was taken aback by my body's response; I had thought that pregnancy was good for my disease, but this time I was wrong. I was prescribed drugs which I was told—to the best of anyone's knowledge—would not cause birth defects. But, in the dark, with fever, Crohn's and the drugs running rampant through my body, I lay awake, filled with dread. Pregnancy had put my health in jeopardy; now my innocent fetus was in danger.

I was fortunate that my disease eventually became quiescent, and I gave birth to a second healthy child. This is not always the case. Each couple must make their own decision whether parenting is worth the risk, and each couple must live with the results of that decision.

Including Your Children When You Are Hospitalized

I was hospitalized for a period of five weeks when my daughter was eighteen months old. I remember how ill I was when I finally agreed to the hospitalization. I put it off as long as possible because I was absolutely convinced that no one would be able to look after her as well as I could. I worried about how to explain to her where I was going. I worried that no one would know when she was sad, that no one would be able to do her hair just right, or that no one would take her to her favorite playground and swing her on her favorite swing. So I hung on, getting weaker, thinner and more ill, until my strength gave out and I had no choice but to go into the hospital.

Because Jack was still training to be a surgeon and frequently had to spend nights on call away from home, my parents took care of our daughter. One night, I received a phone call from my father.

"Ferne," he said, "if Jessica had a fever, how much Tempra would she need?"

I felt helpless. I wanted to be there, but I was physically incapable. I had to learn that someone else was able to care for my child, and that I had to accept the help. I couldn't get used to the idea that I had not abandoned my child or my responsibilities as a mother. When I ultimately came home, we arranged for someone to live in our house. I could get the rest I required and Jessica (and later my two sons Benjamin and Alexander) could stay in their own environment when I required hospitalization. This decision allowed me to feel less guilty about my illness displacing them from the security of their home.

My children understand that their Mommy gets sick. We are always candid about what is going on. We have reinforced many times that my illnes is never their fault. Children often feel responsible when something bad happens to someone they love. They remember all the times they were disciplined and wished you away, and they think that somehow it all came true. This is called magical thought, and is a normal part of a child's emotional development. Because of this potential, it is important to frequently present and reinforce the truth about the parent's illness, and to reassure the children that they are not to blame.

I remember sitting down with Jessica when she was only eighteen months old. We cuddled into a big easy chair. She had her little legs wrapped around my body, and we were face to face. "Jessica," I said, "Mommy has something to tell you that you are not going to like very much. I have to go to the hospital, a big place where people go when they are too sick to take care of themselves anymore. Mommy needs to go there so the doctors and nurses can help her get all better, so we can go to the playground together again. You are going to go and live at Bubbie's house, and she will take very good care of you. She will bring you to see me every day. Once Mommy is better, she will come home again."

The entire time I spoke to her, her eyes did not leave mine. She clung tightly to me as I said good-bye, but she didn't cry. I don't really know how much she understood. Each time she visited with me we repeated the same conversation. This re-enactment, and my words, comforted her. I know that being truthful with my children has been the right thing to do. They know they can believe me whether the news is bad or good.

Sometimes the truth changes and the child will need to be told that a parent has become more ill, even though that parent was expected to get better. It's helpful to discuss how things can sometimes be beyond anyone's control. Children know this from their own experience, but often have trouble applying it to something as awesome as their parent's illness. Simple examples such as a class outing being cancelled because of rain, or having to stay home from school with a cold, may help to make the point.

My husband, parents, in-laws and close friends have always helped to get the children to the hospital to see me. I am convinced that what they see at the hospital will never be as bad as what they see in the depths of their imagination. I can't stress this enough. **Children must be included.** They need to receive accurate information appropriate to their age level. If you are unsure what they can understand, it is better to be concrete and direct.

Children should be taken to visit their parents often. They should also have photos to remind them of the parent they want to see, but can't see as often as they would like. The pictures, cards, scribbles and trinkets that they bring, glowing with pride and affection, have a positive healing effect on the ill parent. They should be displayed in a conspicuous part of the hospital room, so that the children see them when they come to visit, and know that they are valued for their contribution. The hospital room should have a special place for the child to leave some treasured activities and belongings, so that there is a secure place in an otherwise hostile environment.

Children should never be deprived of their parent just because there are tubes or other gadgets running in and out of the parent's body. A child's imagination is an incredible thing, and it can create a far bigger monster than medical science ever will. When children envision intravenous tubing from its description, and then finally see the actual device, they are usually relieved to see how small it really is.

The most important thing a child wants to know is:

"Does it hurt?" Whenever my children ask me this question—and they ask it often—I am always truthful. I calmly tell them that if it did hurt I would look as if I were in pain. I then ask them if I look as if I am in pain. If I don't, they will be able to tell, and will completely relax. If something hurts I will tell them, and will ask that they kiss it for me and make it feel better. Sometimes they will ask a nurse to do something to help the hurt go away. Children are concerned with pain because it is something they have experienced themselves. They are protective of their parent and don't want their parent to suffer. By encouraging children to help, you are allowing them to become involved with your illness. They feel a part of it, rather than estranged from you. As Jessica and Benjamin get older, they try to do some of the things that I do for them when they are ill. It is normal for children to imitate their parents, and it is a source of comfort for the parent to see themselves reflected in their child's kindness.

During one hospitalization, Benjamin and Jessica came to see me. Jessica was very comfortable with the whole experience, but Benjamin was not as seasoned. After casing the room, he started to case me. He focused on my IV and insisted on having his little hands wrapped in adhesive tape, too. After the visit was over, he proudly marched down the hallway, waving his taped hands for everyone to see. At home, Jack could not convince him to take the tape off. Somehow he had maintained his connection with me through the tape on his hands. It was his way of holding onto a piece of his Mommy, even though he had to leave her behind.

Giving your children a necklace, a scarf or any article of your clothing can help them feel secure that you are still with them when you cannot be. If you are accustomed to reading stories to your children at bedtime, make a tape of their favorite ones so that they can play it before bed and fall asleep with your voice in their heads. To this day, my daughter still sleeps with a stuffed bear that I gave to her during my first hospitalization, and she still remembers the day I gave it to her.

The staff at your child's school or day care should be kept up-to-date, so that they can observe and support the child during this time of stress. A school psychologist's help may be necessary for particularly lengthy or devastating reactions to parent illnesses. Jessica had a wonderful teacher in nursery school. The teacher called me often so that I could keep abreast of Jessica's reaction to my illness and how it affected her at school. This was her first "real" school experience, and the teachers often found her staring out the window with tears in her eyes. They would cuddle her, or engage her in one of her favorite activities. The local librarian was consulted to choose books for her that were specifically written for children coping with hospitalization and illness.

Jessica felt as lonesome for me as I did for her. I let her know how much I missed her. It's important to let your child know your feelings. Children are very perceptive, and can tell more from your body language than you imagine. By sharing your feelings with them, you give them licence to share their feelings with you. Sadness away from each other is the depth of loneliness; the sharing of that sadness provides immeasurable comfort to you both.

There are as many issues surrounding partnership and children as there are people with chronic illness. The unique dynamics of each family change the priorities up and down the list. But sharing your feelings, and being truthful with the ones you love are essential for getting through rough spots and surviving daily battles.

Once you make the decision to become involved in a relationship or have a family, you take on a lifelong responsibility. You must care for them, you must protect them from harm, you must love them and you must allow them to always be part of your life, particularly when you are ill.

TWELVE

Loneliness and Alienation

It is very difficult to describe the kind of loneliness experienced by a person with chronic illness. It is not the kind that goes away after talking about it in the wee hours of the night or after a wonderful evening with friends or family. The symptoms of the illness take you out of the mainstream of life, leaving you intensely lonely. Webster's dictionary defines "alone" as "by oneself; solitary; lonesome; standing apart from others of its kind; isolated." Ah, isolation, now we're getting somewhere.

All of these feelings, and the concept of isolation, just begin to describe how people with chronic illness feels from the moment they have symptoms that make them "different" from other people. As members of society, we all observe trends, and we all obey the social rules dictating what is and what is not accepted or valued. It takes very little time to figure out that severe diarrhea, pain and fatigue are not trendsetting distinctions.

The emotional pain the illness inflicts, as well as the daily rituals we undertake and the disasters we prepare for, sets us apart from the rest of the world. The world doesn't seem to know or care about our needs—at least, it seems that way when after walking for miles there is still no access to a public bathroom. Is it fair that a sick person has to buy some food in a restaurant in order to have the privilege of using a bathroom?

Once I received an invitation from a new friend to go out for dinner with family members who were visiting from out of town. Just before we left, my bowels started acting up. Jack asked me if he should call our friends and cancel the plans. It had been a long time since I had gone out for a meal with people who didn't know about my Crohn's disease. I feared having to excuse myself for the numerous trips to the bathroom and facing the inquisitive glances. I hated putting Jack in the position of explaining my absence from the table. (At least I have developed radar and can find a woman's room in any location in under ten seconds!) I reminded myself how close friends reassured me that I always felt more aware of the absences than they did. I decided that I didn't want us to miss the chance for an enjoyable evening.

What a mistake! My gut started to do its twisting dance even before the meal was served. By the time we were halfway through dinner I had made two more trips to the bathroom. Our host for the evening commented that the restaurant must have a wonderful restroom since I seemed to want to see it so often. I laughed along with everyone else, and secretly weighed the options of telling versus not telling. If I didn't tell, he would not get the facts straight. If I did tell, he might feel uncomfortable that he had made a joke about a serious medical condition. I was in a bind. Although Crohn's disease is not socially acceptable mealtime conversation, I did not want my host to think I was a Drug Addict using the privacy of the restroom to get a fix. I decided to explain briefly and humorously asked the people at the table to carry on without me, if necessary. I just wanted to go home but feared that I would hurt my friend's feelings and ruin yet another evening for Jack. That night as we drove home in the car I felt miserable. All I could think about was how different and alone I felt.

Pain behind the closed door of a bathroom is a very lonely experience. As the sweat pours down your brow, you wonder if there will ever be a day you won't feel like this. You are alone, and you know that no one can do anything to change it.

When the doctor announces that you have Crohn's disease, your family and friends rally to support you. When the lights go out at night and the day is over (either in a hospital room or in your own cozy bed at home), you are alone in the dark with that knowledge. No amount of support and compassion, hand-holding or hugging will ever take away that kind of loneliness. During some very awful moments, when I didn't think I could face one more moment of pain, my mother has told me, "I only wish I could bear this for you." She wants to help me. She wants to take the disease away and protect me from the pain and suffering. She does not want me to bear this suffering by myself. But when she leaves my bedside, I still have to face it alone. Living with chronic illness takes strength that I am not always certain I have.

What can help us face this sense of isolation and loneliness, so we can continue our day-to-day existence without experiencing such tremendous emotional pain? This is neither a simple question nor a straightforward task. Everyone has unique methods of coping or not coping with stress. However, most human beings seek each other out for company and support. This is the best emotional medicine.

Join a group such as the Crohn's and Colitis Foundation of Canada (CCFC) or the Crohn's and Colitis Foundation of America (CCFA). There are similar self-help groups for most chronic illnesses. Look them up in your telephone book. These organizations may be a good starting point for many people, and they provide many types of supportive activities for both the sufferer and the family. There are educational meetings and social events that allow people with the same problem to meet one another in an atmosphere of acceptance and familiarity. It is comforting to be able to speak freely in a situation where you are not alone with your disease. The challenge is to hold on to this feeling of community and strength, and use it to combat the ongoing loneliness in your daily life.

Not all people feel at ease in large groups; nor do all people want to share their story with strangers. The CCFC and CCFA try to send people who are comfortable with their illness, to visit sufferers in hospital, to help them make contact with their new community.

If you are not comfortable with organized "coping," turn to the people around you for support. I have been approached many times by parents, in-laws, spouses and other concerned individuals about the sufferer they love but don't know how to support. But isn't that feeling really the main issue? By finding a person who loves you and is motivated to share your experience, you already feel less alone. Family members often find themselves in the active role of supporter, but they themselves need support. Sometimes questions that they are afraid to ask or issues that they are afraid to confront are easier to explore when they talk to a person with the disease. I have received phone calls from family members and friends asking me to help clarify what their loved one is experiencing. They know the person and I know the disease. Between us, a greater understanding is reached. There are many people in the chronic illness community who offer this type of lay support. It is just a matter of finding them.

Some people with chronic illness cope best by isolating themselves from the world during a flare-up, and ignoring their illness when it is in remission. They flit back and forth between the "normal" world and the "sick" world. Although this is a common situation, they carry a secret burden around with them year after year. Eventually, it becomes impossible to keep the two worlds apart; they overlap, and a crisis ensues. I am not saying that we are defined by our illness, but we must recognize that it is as much a part of us as our hair color, stature, and personality.

Once you have accepted your illness as a part of you, and have tried to live within its limitations, you will find that you become increasingly more comfortable with letting the rest of the world in on your secret. From this acceptance, you will derive the courage and energy to combat the loneliness and seek support. These are the first steps to bridging the gap between you and the surrounding world.

This does not mean that the days of coveting other

people's health will be over. Every time you feel alone with your illness, you may still want to crumple up in a corner or jump off the roof. You have to learn how to accept these emotions and find understanding people to support you. Learn to cultivate relationships that reinforce your ability to talk about and face your feelings. Try to spend time with people who accept your illness as part of you. Remember that there will be days when you feel so alone that you cannot accept that there is a person in the world who feels as bad as you do. It's hard to believe, but feeling this way can be a very therapeutic experience. The "nobody knows the trouble I've seen" feeling is the bottom and the only place you can go from there is up. Self-pity can be healing. Once you've picked yourself up and brushed yourself off, you will emerge feeling nurtured and stronger.

Seek out others and recognize the power that their support gives you. Whether you choose a self-help organization, counseling services in your medical or religious community, or your family and friends, these people will help you feel strong enough to take the first steps toward reaching out and ending the loneliness.

THIRTEEN

Hospitalization and Health-Care Providers

Going to the Emergency Room

The times I seem to feel the most sorry for myself, and have the time to ask the unanswerable question of my lifetime, "Why me?" is when I am admitted to the hospital. So much has been written on the dehumanizing experience of institutional life that I will not take the time to bore you with that. Let's just say that there are very few experiences that will take place during your chronic illness career which are like hospitalization.

Many chronically ill are hospitalized on an emergency basis. When the pain of partial bowel obstruction begins, my heart pounds furiously. This intense reaction is in anticipation of the admission procedure I know I'll face at the entrance to the emergency department. If this takes place early in the morning, and my physician is unavailable, I contend with having to triage myself. Triage is what medical people do to determine how severe your problem is and it allows them to decide who is in dire need of immediate attention.

If you choose to call your doctor's office first, the secretary or nurse will most likely ask you, "Is this an emergency?" The standard tone of voice implies that, of course, it isn't. Phrased in this way, it is an intimidating question and very few of us feel comfortable giving ourselves full marks—despite how badly we feel. As a consequence, you re-examine and then downplay your symptoms. You know you've been up all night with severe pain and nausea but, inwardly, you really want someone to confirm that it will go away without medical intervention. We all know what's awaiting us at the hospital, we simply want to delay the inevitable rather than face up to the urgency of the problem.

Unless you are vomiting your guts out, bleeding profusely, unable to move or have a temperature hovering in the sizzling range, you might even be inclined to answer, "Well, I'm not quite sure." While you say these words into the mouthpiece, your mind reruns the previous evening's events, which led to this phone call. In spite of being up most of the night with pain, you now agree to wait until the doctor can get back to you. If I had been keeping score, I'd say it was Secretary: 1, Patient: 0. Know and accept that these people have been trained in the fine art of intimidation.

Many physicians actually instruct their receptionists to guard them by using these tactics. One physician admitted to me that the secretary who works in his office is familiar with certain regulars (patients who know the ropes). They tell the secretary what they need. This means that the less frequent patients who don't know the ropes do not receive the same treatment. It also means that receptionists need guidance from you. You need to learn how to tell them when you need help. They have been programmed to separate the needy patient from the patient who regularly and needlessly consults with doctors. Unfortunately, these patients tend to be more persistent, whereas we usually back off at the first sign of resistance. Don't back off!

After you've established that you need to be seen urgently, it's off to the emergency department. Once there, your chart will be collected and you will be kept waiting. Unless you're lucky enough to have your physician call ahead, this stage can take anywhere from thirty minutes to four hours or longer. The length of time depends on how busy the emergency department is. When your name is finally called, you are led down a hallway and placed in a stark room that is often divided with flimsy curtains into cubicles that are supposed to provide privacy. Through them, you can see and hear everything imaginable so privacy is not really what is accomplished. This is an introduction to the dehumanizing experience yet to come. It's a good idea to bring a supportive person to keep you company and buoy your spirits in preparation for the long haul.

Next, you see the intern. As he or she gazes at the chart—which is clearly marked, Part 13 (out of 13)—the intern may then ask you the most comical question of the century: "Have you ever been in hospital before?" For a moment you pause, look at the intern, and think, "Naw, she really didn't ask me that." You look into the intern's eyes and realize she is actually serious. You sigh, lean forward and wish you had a copy of that printed sheet, which you keep threatening to make, that details your Crohn's Career. (This, by the way, is an excellent idea.) Even the obvious can sometimes be obscured by the custodians.

The procedures ahead range from simple X-rays and blood tests to flexible sigmoidoscopies. Depending on your chronic illness, you will get a chance to become reacquainted with old, familiar tests. Whenever the emergency room nurses see me coming, they run the other way. They know that one of them will most likely have to start my intravenous and none of them are ever ready to face my difficult veins. You would think that whoever created my body would have had the foresight to give me good veins, if he knew I would need them so badly.

If you already have an established relationship with a doctor, are feeling poorly and you are not in the mood for the numerous rectal exams and other sundry tests, which are often performed in the name of medical education, **you can refuse the treatment by a doctor-in-training**. Sometimes I think I should be sent a commendation for all the medical students my body has personally helped train. Yet even the most seasoned veterans of the emergency department will find themselves uncomfortable about refusing medical "treatment" from doctors in training. You are your own keeper and no one should make you feel guilty for asserting yourself. We don't always have the patience to be "good" patients and, in the sometimes frenetic world of modern medicine, the patient has to look out for his or her own best interests.

After all this, and once you've established that you will be taking a room at the inn, relax. It's always at least three hours before they can find a bed for you.

Being Admitted

I always sense a ghost when I'm admitted to a new hospital room: the ghost of everything I have missed because I was too sick to attend. A sadness wells up from deep inside me while I watch people from my bed. They come into my room and tell me, secondhand, what is going on in the outside world. I depend on this lifeline. It allows me to feel in touch with normal, everyday existence. Is it hot outside? Cold? Being in a climate-controlled setting stops you from being able to know the joy of wind on your face, or the need for a raincoat.

I share a piece of my life with them, and they with me. I feel so sad when the exchange is over, and they wish me well as they leave. They go back out into the world, where life goes on. I'm left in the vacuum of the institutional world, where life and time seem warped. You're never exactly sure what day or time it is except by looking at the activities going on. There is no place to escape from these activities. Whether you are hungry or not, dinner may arrive as early as 4:30 in the afternoon. You are dependent on your custodians to feed you—so, hungry or not, you eat. They decide when you sleep, urinate, move your bowels, get dressed and even visit with friends. You aren't allowed many independent decisions.

There are days when I feel depressed by the sameness of it all. The routines and the illness are some days just too much to bear. On those days, I conjure up a memory. There is a place in my mind where I preserve memories of particularly pleasing or amusing events, scenes, interactions and other aspects of life experiences that I keep close to my heart. I call this my "mind box of memories." I started this collection a long time ago when I was first hospitalized and had lengthy periods away from common social interaction. During these periods, night turns to day because of lack of sleep, and too much idle time feeds an active mind. Thinking only about being sick can get boring. Breaking away and "playing" something peaceful or funny creates a good change of pace, like your own video machine. Music often helps me enter my memory box, and I never go into the hospital without a radio or cassette player.

Some people turn to soap operas, others to romance novels or crossword puzzles. I like to read and knit. No matter what diversion you choose, it will remind you that life is more than white coats, dull days, pain, discomfort and sadness.

While I am in the hospital, visiting me becomes an activity for some people during their lunch hour. After a few visits, however, most of them find other, more amusing pastimes. My close friends and family drop many of their responsibilities to spend time supporting me, and the traveling back and forth to the "inn" eventually becomes a tremendous burden. For many reasons, after a while, the visitors mostly stop.

I'm not foolish enough to think that I have done anything wrong to cause this: I recognize that everyone has their own life and responsibilities. My room, once filled with flowers, has barely a single rose. It's not that people have stopped caring. It's simply that your illness is a part of you now. People expect you to be hospitalized. People expect you to come home. People expect that you are used to being in the hospital, and that they don't need to pay attention to it anymore.

Our visitors are our lifeline to the outside world. They help to break up the institutional boredom, change the pace, and most of all increase our self-image and boost our ego. We need to know that we are still considered active members of society. We fear being treated as if we no longer exist and that our presence does not even make a ripple in life's pond. You may find yourself becoming disappointed with certain people, family and friends, as there is no evidence of them at your bedside and in your mailbox. You are astounded at the inconsiderate behavior and wonder why they can't take the few minutes away from their coveted, healthy life to send you a card, or call or visit. How do you forgive these friends when you see them happily walking down the street on a sunny day, with their family in tow, ice cream cones in hand, and seemingly not a care in the world? And, later, how do you respond to their inquiries into your health? If you carry around these hurts, they become a heavy burden. After years, the load will become monstrous, and will demand energy you can't spare. I am hurt at times, but if those feelings linger, they drain precious energy that is better spent elsewhere.

There is a part of you that may not be able to forgive your absent friends. Through experiences like these, you learn how important it is to have a reliable partner or loyal family members or friends, because they are your core support. They are with you for the long haul. They are your nucleus.

Nurses, Doctors-in-Training, Social Workers and Physiotherapists

There are many care-givers in the hospital, but nurses have the greatest potential to be supportive and make you comfortable during those long days and nights. If they put their training to good use, they can actively support your family and friends, and be a strong advocate and bridge between you and the workings of the hospital. Since I am a nurse, my testimony will be somewhat biased. On the one hand, I believe good nursing care can be the key to getting better. On the other hand, I have received such a variety of care over the years that I can no longer say this with such assurance. Nurses who work with the chronically ill have a responsibility to take the time to understand what it feels like, to know there is no cure.

Whenever I am admitted to my regular ward, it is like old home week. Past shared experience seems to bond the nurses and chronic illness patients together. But chronic patients also have a great deal of knowledge to impart that may make an inexperienced nurse feel insecure. Such a nurse may feel inadequate and unable to give his or her best. This nurse doesn't share the history I share with the other nurses. My advice to the inexperienced nurse is, don't be put off. I really enjoy having a nurse who is finding out about me for the first time. I may feel more comfortable opening up to him or her during the witching hours of the night. If concern and interest are shown, I am happy to accept the care offered by any nurse, experienced or otherwise.

When I took my first job in nursing, I was assigned to a five-year-old girl who had been chronically ill with kidney failure for six months. One morning, I came into her room carrying a tray with her ten-o'clock medications. She looked into the plastic cup filled almost to the brim with pills. After moving them around with the crook of her little index finger, she announced that I had made a mistake. I had forgotten one of her medications.

I was unaccustomed to being told by a patient that I had made an error, but to be told by a little five-year-old redhead with freckles completely took me by surprise. I looked down at the pills and then at her set jaw. I told her I would be back in a minute and then walked back to the medication room to investigate. Sure enough, she was right! I learned a lot from that little girl. Do not doubt patients who have medical routines as part of their life. They may have a lot to teach you.

Nurses often find that these situations undermine their sense of being in control and make them feel insecure. There must be an open dialogue with patients so that there is a sense of working as a team. If people are working together, there is less tension when something is questioned. The routines that patients have before they come into hospital must be respected. Once they go home, their illness and routines have to go home with them.

There will always be good, bad and mediocre nurses. I often wonder what prompts someone who doesn't really like people to choose this profession. People do strange things. When I was in the hospital recently, I met a real terror. She must have had a bad day. She didn't even try to be pleasant. Jack was visiting in the evening and I was feeling depressed and tired. My right hand was occupied with the intravenous that was giving me fluid until my bowel obstruction subsided. I was only allowed to drink small amounts of water. I picked up the water jug and clumsily spilled the contents on my bed. I rang for the nurse to ask if she could please change my bed. I felt so sick and tired. All I wanted to do was lie down.

I was connected with a ward clerk who told me that my nurse would be there when she got a chance. I waited at the side of my bed. I tried leaning against Jack but the pain was getting worse. Finally I decided that my need to lie down was overwhelming, so I went to the linen room, got some linen and Jack and I made my bed. We were quite a sight, with my hospital gown flapping in the breeze and an intravenous in my hand, as I instructed Jack in the art of hospital bedmaking. My nurse came to the room an hour later with some clean sheets. Jack and I exchanged a look and I told her that I had already remade my bed because it was soaking wet. She was visibly angry.

"Well, I didn't think you'd die waiting in a wet bed," she said, as she turned on her heel and left.

Most people who have been hospitalized have similar stories. What follows is a checklist for nurses to help them know what to do, so that our stories will be full of praise rather than dismay.

A Checklist for Nurses

- Stay and listen when we seem angry or upset. I don't know how many times I wished the nurse would have pushed a little harder so that, with tears running down my face, I could tell her how unfair I thought this illness seemed. Help us pursue our anger and direct it towards a healthier outlet. Help us talk and explore what is bothering us. Our problems may be institution-related, such as inadequate sleep, poor success with getting appropriate food trays, lack of privacy, an incompatible roommate, or a bad experience with an insensitive medical or surgical resident. Nurses are the experts in solving these problems and we require your expertise. Don't forget to inquire what impact the disease is having on our life now. Things are so unpredictabe that what was manageable yesterday may be impossible to handle today.

- Help us by being our true advocates. Stand up for our rights as human beings. Ensure that we get the same treatment you would like your dearest relative to receive. Encourage and teach us to be our own advocates.

- Help shield us from unwanted and excessive visitors. By performing this function, you will help us get the physical and emotional rest we so badly need.

- Become more knowledgeable about our tests so you can really describe them and help allay our fears. Go and see the tests. Talk to us when we come back so that you develop an understanding of what we are really going through when we leave your custody.

- Value and use basic comfort measures such as back rubs with alcohol-based creams to soothe our backs and help us sleep without the ten-o'clock sedative rounds. Darken our rooms, straighten our sheets, comb our hair, wash our furrowed brows. Keep us as pain-free as possible. Try to believe that we really are suffering. Encourage your institution to give painkillers by intravenous routes rather than by intramuscular

injections, because we don't need any additional sour-
ces of pain. Try to anticipate our needs so that we can
feel as close to being ourselves as is humanly possible.
- Give us independence, but not so much that we feel
  we have all the responsibility for getting well.
- Help our families by communicating our progress to
  them and by being their advocate as well.

Your job is an important one, and if you wish to take
it on, we promise to work with you to get as well as
we possibly can.

FOURTEEN

Changing Your Life's Direction

Some people are diagnosed with chronic illness very early on and learn to set realistic goals and expectations from the start. For the rest of us, who are innocently expecting life to unfold as it should, the diagnosis is like a head-on collision. The casualties are numerous and they often include your life-plan.

In the past, you were rewarded for your efforts, and found that hard work and perseverence allowed you to achieve your goals. "If I want something, I play by the rules and I will succeed." That was me. Unfortunately for all of us, those are not the rules of chronic illness.

Everyone is susceptible to chronic illness—good people, bad people, deserving people and not-so-deserving people all can get sick. If you believe strongly in fate, you might think that chronic illness will lead your life along a path that would otherwise not have been taken, as if it was the way your life was meant to go. If you are not a fatalist, you may have more difficulty in viewing the changes positively. Having to alter a childhood dream may be more than you will be able to bear, along with the other responsibilities and losses thay your illness imposes on you. But no matter how you feel about it, there is no question that your life's direction will be altered by your disease.

Choosing a career when you have chronic illness can be very tricky. Since ileitis and colitis are commonly diagnosed in the teens or early adulthood, many of us are in the process of educating ourselves towards careers when the illness parachutes into our lives. Sometimes illness and education become incompatible. Like a bad marriage, the wrong career choice can destroy your remaining health. It can place so much weight on your life that the foundation finally collapses. Even if your education or training is complete, you may need to consider a career change. Consulting with a career counsellor might help you move laterally and preserve the aspects of your career you want without the deadly stress.

A job with strict deadlines, huge time demands, late hours or one in which one person is indispensable, can be disastrous for healthy people. To combine these types of jobs with a chronic illness can be deadly.

When I started my first full-time job, my illness had been in remission for about eighteen months. I was feeling well. Being a staff nurse in a pediatric hospital was very demanding both emotionally and physically. I loved giving the children the sensitivity I felt I had missed during some of my own hospitalizations. I became focused on helping the children and their families cope with the pain of illness, and I worked very hard. The twelve-hour night shift put a quick end to my remission. After six months, I applied for a job that involved strictly day and evening shifts.

I knew I that if I could not get that job, I would have to quit. I explained my situation in detail to the head nurse when I applied for the new position. I was fortunate that she understood and respected the circumstances.

Prior to taking a job, talk to your potential employer about your physical limitations. You don't have to label yourself a "sick" person immediately, but the issue of health will come up during the interview. If it happens to be skipped over, you shouldn't necessarily breathe a sigh of relief—almost all establishments will ask you to take an employee health exam. If you aren't candid about a major health problem, the examining physician will be the bearer of this news. The person who hired you may worry that this is something you deliberately covered up or, worse, lied about.

In my discussions with potential employers, I usually wait until I know that I'm interested in the job, and sense that they are interested in me. Once this is established, I make it a rule never to leave without initiating a discussion of my limitations as a future employee. I stress how productive I am when well, and emphasize the sensitivity that I bring to my work. I've learned that no job is worth sacrificing my health, and that revealing my illness and its limitations to my employer after I've been offered the job traps them unfairly.

Never take advantage of sick-time. Using up those mental-health days may leave you short when your illness acts up. On the other hand, don't overcompensate. If you are ill, stay home. People with chronic illness can get a virus during flu season, just like everyone else.

If you do decide to change jobs because the demands are too great, you may find help from employment agencies specializing in career changes. In the best case scenario, your ex-employer will be understanding and make some arrangements for you during this difficult period. Financial concerns play an important role in pushing us beyond our bodies' limitations. If you are the main breadwinner in your family or you are supporting yourself, you may have to apply for unemployment insurance. Unfortunately, fewer financial resources, especially if you feel you are to blame, can weigh heavily on your shoulders.

Disability insurance, if acquired before your diagnosis, may see you through these difficult times. If they are able, don't hesitate to call for help from family and friends.

No matter how much support you have, changing jobs because of illness is an unenviable position to be in. But choosing to remain in a job that is destructive to your health is worse: you may lose your remaining health and you could still lose the job, anyway.

Perhaps this is an opportunity to extricate yourself from a job that you have had a long-standing ambivalence about, or an opportunity to try something you never had the nerve to try before. I remember talking to a twenty-two-year-old man who was hospitalized for bowel rest and receiving nutrition through a nasogastric tube. He told me how guilty he felt for not working at his construction job with his father and uncle, the way he had every summer since he was fifteen. Ill for years, he'd always managed; this was the first summer he hadn't been able to cope. After talking for a while and commiserating with him about the unfairness of chronic illness, he shyly admitted that he'd always wanted to be a lawyer but was afraid his family wouldn't feel comfortable about this career choice. Crohn's disease may have provided the impetus he needed to pursue a change in his life's direction.

Sometimes changes come too fast and furiously—giving up a career, accepting a diagnosis, putting up with medications and their side effects, learning new family roles—are more than we can tolerate. Psychological or spiritual help through these intense times may be extremely helpful.

Career Checklist

If you are considering training for an occupation or changing jobs, ask yourself these questions:
1) Can I physically cope with the expectations of this job/training?
2) What will I have to give up to do this job/training adequately?
3) Will this job/training compromise my health any further?
4) What are the anticipated long-term effects of this job/training on me? On my family?
5) Does my partner support my decision to do this? Will this job/training increase his or her level of stress?

I had a friend who was a twenty-one-year-old medical student when he was diagnosed with Crohn's disease. The symptoms had plagued him for a long time. As he entered the final year of medical school, his hours became erratic and the disease flared up more frequently. He was always tired and the prednisone gave him incredible mood swings. Before entering medical school, he'd entertained the idea of becoming a cardiovascular surgeon. Two of his family members were surgeons and he had assumed his training would take him in this direction.

As his internship year approached, he was hospitalized

intermittently for various complications of the disease. The pain and exhaustion were making it more and more difficult to drag himself to the hospital each day. His internship year began on a surgical rotation. After two weeks of long hours, no sleep, extreme preparation demands for rounds and long hours standing on his feet, he was admitted to the hospital with a bowel obstruction. During this setback he resolved, with the help of the staff psychologist, to direct himself to an area of specialty with fewer physical demands. By choosing another specialty in the field of medicine, he was able to utilize his years of study and not give up everything.

To realistically incorporate chronic illness into your life, you can choose a career that is interesting and stimulating, yet still within your physical capabilities. Often it may not be what you originally planned. If you have to give up a career filled with excitement or prestige, which for some people is a bitter pill to swallow, try and compensate by focusing on, and enhancing, other activities you enjoy. (By beating the career issue into the ground, you will have put all your energy into flogging a horse that is already dead.) List things you always said you would do if only you had the time. If your list includes music, browse through brochures and buy tickets for a concert series, or follow radio schedules and set aside time for listening. Watch for free concerts at local parks and shopping centers. Make a list of books you want to read and rummage through used bookstores to find them. Join a workout studio or exercise class at a local community center to enjoy when your energy level is high. Go for long walks, and spend more time talking to your partner.

Keep the list in a place where you can refer to it often. Reward yourself for completing what you set out to do by treating yourself to a coffee, lunch or dinner, or a new something you've been wanting. Don't look at career accomplishments as the only valid rewards. Take the opportunity and time to focus elsewhere.

It's important to realize that your chronic illness may prevent you from ever winning the Nobel prize or the Boston Marathon. Once you've dealt with the anger and frustration of not realizing a particular goal, move forward by refocusing and adjusting your career decisions. Seeking rewards elsewhere will ultimately provide you with a fuller and healthier life.

FIFTEEN

This Time the Decision was Mine

It took me over five years to make the decision to have another ileostomy. Of all the suffering that my illness has brought me over the years, this decision was the most painful because I knew it was permanent. Once I made it, I could never go back.

A wise surgeon once told me that he always recognizes patients who have come to a decision on their own. They enter his office with their "hat in their hand," asking for the arrangements to be made for their surgery. I've always pictured this as a person waving white flags; someone who has surrendered to their illness. I resolved that I would never be that person. I would never enter a surgeon's office with my hat in my hand.

Five years of constant hospitalizations, pain and alteration of my life beyond recognition almost brought me to my knees. One morning, I went shopping for food with my children. I had used the bathroom moments before leaving for the expedition, but as I trudged down the very first aisle, my abdomen was gripped with pain. My son was in the upper part of the cart, and my daughter was gliding along beside it. Neither was aware of the impending crisis.

I knew that I would have to leave them to make that familiar, hated beeline to the bathroom. Taking them along would use up precious seconds. I quickly instructed my daughter to wait and keep watch over her brother.

"What if somebody comes Mommy?" she said with noticeable panic.

"Scream as loudly as you can," I said, and dashed away.

On my return, I found them engaged in counting all the loaves of bread on the shelf. All was well with them, but not with me. I knew I could no longer go to a public place with them if we weren't accompanied by another adult.

The voice of my surgeon, who I had resented for so long, entered my head: "If you have the ileostomy, you will feel better. You will get off your drugs. You won't be dependent on bathrooms."

But what would that mean? Bowel obstructions every month, for ten months. Constant skin irritations and unalleviated itching so bad I would want to scratch off the entire top layer of my skin. The embarrassment of having a piece of red bowel sticking out of the front of my belly. What about being physically different? Would my kids be disgusted? Would my husband reject me? Would I reject myself? Could I face friends and family? Would I want to live after that kind of surgery?

These were the questions I had repeatedly asked myself during the past year. And the answers had never supported a decision to have "the operation." I entertained the idea that maybe I didn't want to get well. Maybe I liked being sick? The next night, at four a.m., I lay sweating while my belly cramped. I had woken for the fifth time since I had turned in at eleven. Exhausted, I realized that my body was making my decision for me.

The final showdown, I less-than-fondly remember, was actually an accumulation of events. I had developed fevers that raged through my body each day. I couldn't tolerate food and what I did eat made such a quick trip through my bowel I shouldn't have bothered. I was unable to go more than forty-five minutes at a time without cramps disrupting my sleep. I was yelling at my precious children whenever they didn't do as they were told. I no longer had any energy. I feared my husband's touch. Everything hurt.

Finally, one night, I decided to try on the idea of "the surgery." I was lying in a hot bath, something I did constantly to get relief from pain. My husband came into the bathroom and I asked him, "If I had an ileostomy again, how would you feel?" He turned to me and said, "If it would make you feel better, then I think you should go for it."

In the ensuing conversation, we tried to answer all the dreaded questions that had lurked in my head and heart for five long years. Would he find my body disgusting? What should we tell the children? Will they reject me? If this was permanent, and I had problems like the last time, what would I do? I threatened suicide if I was trapped in a life of bowel obstructions, nasogastric tubes and pain. By the time our conversation ended, my skin was as wrinkled as a prune. It dawned on me, then, that I was already trapped—I was sacrificing my young adulthood and no longer had any freedom. My disease had brought me to a crossroad. Rather than view the ileostomy as my enemy, something to surrender to, I realized suddenly that surgery was my bid for freedom.

A week later, I sat in my surgeon's office with my hat in my hand. I had informed him over the telephone how ill I was and that I needed to talk with him.

"I have decided to have an ileostomy."

"Are you sure?" he asked. "Maybe you should give it more thought."

"I have been thinking about this for five years and I don't need to think about it any more. If the operation has a possibility of giving me back my life, then lets just do it," I said.

Within hours, I was in the land of doctors, nurses and blood-letting technicians, each wanting a part of me. Like a child who wants to bypass the boring parts of a story, I wanted to skip all these tests and procedures. The surgery, however, went fine and, despite some major setbacks, I eventually got to the end of the story.

I can now state with confidence that this was a good decision. At the best of times, having an ileostomy is not perfect. But I only had an array of imperfect, negative choices: a life of imprisonment from the symptoms of the disease, or a life with body-altering surgery that I may never come to terms with. I had tried the jail term and I wanted to be released.

I recently discussed these options with a pre-adolescent girl who also felt trapped by her illness. She had the same array of negative choices. In helping her make a decision, I told her about the lists we all make in our heads of things we want to do. They include everything from short-term desires such as wanting to eat an ice cream sundae to long-term goals such as deciding on a career or getting rid of your disease.

When you have to consider your illness before anything else in life, you feel trapped and angry. Over time, the list of things to do for your disease gets longer, and the list of exciting things to do for yourself shrinks. The scale is tipped and life begins to feel like a compromise; soon, you feel like you have lost all control. At this point, you are simply surviving. If these words describe you, it may be time to seriously reconsider the alternatives.

The ileostomy gave me back some control over my life. Although it's still not perfect, I can now plan things with some assurance that they will happen, and make decisions without first having to consider the Crohn's beast.

SIXTEEN

Getting Better—
The Ultimate Control

What does it mean to get better?

If you were to ask various people with chronic illness what their most important long-term goal is, you would hear a unanimous, resounding, "To Get Better!" This is the dream of the chronically ill.

Being sick is a universal experience. Most people recover and return to lives pretty much untouched by their illness. This is not the case for the person with chronic illness. No matter how many times we "get better," we will more often than not become sick again. Unable to plan for it, we know it is inevitable and we await it with dread.

After my last surgery, I felt extremely well and I no longer had to cope with ongoing pain and other debilitating symptoms. At first, the realization and sensation made me giddy and carefree. I was in love: smitten with health. I had so much energy, and no longer felt tired and defeated at the end of each day. But as I charged forward towards my new life, a strange thing happened— I started to feel depressed and directionless. I was almost paralyzed by my new energy. I became confused, until I realized what was happening. I didn't know how to live now that I was *better*!

My life had changed. I no longer felt like a lifetime member of "the club." Did I really belong to the Healthy People Club now? I'd been sick for so long, I couldn't remember the rules or etiquette. I'm not sure I ever knew them. All the energy I had previously devoted to coping with pain symptoms and disappointment was now available to me, but I couldn't seem to put it to good use. What was the matter with me?

All my adult life, I had lived with an image of myself that was shaped by my illness. My relationships with people often revolved around my illness. The way I planned my life and the way I looked at life was colored by my illness. Now I was changing. I was someone very different. Outwardly, I was the same. My name had not changed, even my everyday activities had not changed. Something as powerful as an earthquake had shaken my foundation and the dust was settling in a different pattern.

This scenario can happen to anyone. One day we go to the doctor and he tells us the nightmare is over.

During the war with illness we meet others in the same situation who become our allies. They teach us to cope. They become our friends, our support and sometimes even our family. Not having to explain, knowing that they understand how you feel, gives you comfort. How can healthy people possibly understand?

When you get better, you aren't part of the group anymore. You are banished to live among the "healthy people" now and you feel lost without your old allies but you can't take them with you because they are still involved with the fight. It is suddenly very lonely.

Getting better is like growing up. When I was constantly sick, my key support people were thrust into the role of protector. All my suffering created a relationship built on dependency. When I got better, I no longer needed protection. Like an adolescent, I wanted to breathe as an adult and make adult decisions, be able to crash and pick up the pieces by myself. Despite my impatience for freedom, my parents held on tightly to their role—we all knew the stakes were high.

Learning to be healthy is almost as difficult as learning to be sick. The rules change and you have to find out what the rules mean for you. If your parents, spouse or friend protected you, they will need a chance to get used to the new you. We've had longer to work out the changes and are impatient to get on with our new lives. We want to try out our new wings. Our protectors and supporters need time to catch up. We must be sensitive to how our change in health affects them. It is possible that getting better creates some difficulties for them. They may not feel as needed or loved.

Some people thrive on control and may choose a mate based on his or her dependency. By getting better, we completely alter the dynamics in a marriage—or any relationship. These changes and effects need to be discussed openly and honestly. This may be the time to seek help from friends or a professional.

Independence—and reorganization: we missed this part of growing up by being sick. Change is scary for everyone, but once it happens you will have finally completed the part of your life that your illness stole from you.

SEVENTEEN

A Word From the Spouse

I still remember the way Ferne looked the first time I met her. We were sixteen years old, both starting work at summer camp, both excited about the end of school and the beginning of an adventure. She was standing on the swim dock in a bikini, with her hair blond and frizzy and wild in the wind. There was an aura of youthfulness and freedom around her. At five foot two and 95 pounds, she struck me as a tiny bundle of energy, cute, feisty and confident.

We became friends over that summer, and spent the following year—our final year of high school—extricating ourselves from other relationships. When I went away to university, we carried on a long-distance relationship. She complained periodically about bellyaches, and slowly lost what little weight she had. She had tests (all normal) and carried on, ignoring the signals her body was giving her. I tried to support her but found myself thinking privately that it must be all in her head. This was partly because I assumed that doctors knew what they were talking about (an assumption I now know to be wrong quite often), but also, and more importantly, because I didn't want there to be anything wrong.

That spring, on the day Ferne finished her final exam, her endurance ran out. Her mother drove her from her exam to the hospital, and within a day she was being operated on. The next week was a blur of white coats, intravenous drips, hushed hallway conversations and furrowed brows. But the most vivid image in my mind is Ferne's face; in it was a mixture of fear, pain and helplessness. I didn't understand much of what was said, words like "megacolon," "nasogastric tube" and "ileostomy" were thrown about, each one more sinister than the last. When the decision was made to proceed with an ileostomy, Ferne was terrified that I would abandon her. She clung to me even to the point of excluding her parents. I repeatedly watched the door close, blocking out the hurt expression on their faces. They said they were happy Ferne had someone so supportive, but deep inside I felt they didn't quite trust me. Perhaps it was because I didn't quite trust myself.

Although I knew that most boys my age would have made an excuse and taken off, I couldn't. I had no control over the course of events, but I could at least provide some support for Ferne and her family. Just being there, holding her hand or watching her sleep off the morphine, was a visible act of support. I wondered how the spunky, independent girl I met on the swim dock had turned into such a terribly sick, frightened person, and all I wanted was for that healthy girl to come back. Reassuring her fifteen or twenty times a day that she would still be attractive to me, that I would still want to be with her, seemed to be all she wanted. I wasn't sure if I believed it myself, but I intended to give it my best shot.

As time went on she felt better, and the dynamics changed. First she started complaining about the food, the nurses, the bathroom facilities. Then she started in on her doctors: they didn't visit often enough, or for long enough. They treated her gruffly or ignored her. I certainly wasn't immune: I arrived late, I didn't bring flowers, I looked too interested when a pretty nurse walked by. It was hard to take this kind of criticism. After all, hadn't I just sacrificed my whole summer for her? Wasn't I the best goddamn boyfriend the world had ever seen? I got sick of the complaining, and at times, dreading the thought of another visit, would go AWOL. Guilt usually brought me back to endure another round.

Through the years, the disease has relentlessly pursued its course. It hides, quiescent, until we relax a bit, and then it strikes with fury. It presents itself in diverse ways, catching us off guard and confusing even the most astute of doctors. During remissions, we convince ourselves that life is finally normal, and with each flare-up we revert to our old patterns and adopt our old postures. Ferne stops eating, begins to lose weight and complains of pain and fevers. We wonder what is happening. Is it the flu? Maybe a mild bowel obstruction or something she ate. She asks me what I think.

"I don't want to be your doctor," I say. "Why don't you call Dr. X?"

"What can he possibly tell me?" she says.

When she finally crashes and hospitalization is inevitable, it is as if we've both failed. I didn't get her there early enough, didn't push hard enough. I kick myself for giving in to her denial. She feels that she failed because she got sick again. She is convinced that this would never have happened if she had eaten better, been more compliant with her medication, or pushed herself a little less hard at work. People who feel guilty make lousy partners, and we each struggle to behave "appropriately." I act strong and supportive and she plays the role of the good patient.

But then the undercurrent of anger at her disease, which threatens to surface day in and day out, breaks through and erupts like a volcano. But at whom can she direct her anger? The doctors aren't around enough (although they certainly take a verbal beating out of earshot), the children are too innocent and she is afraid of alienating her friends. The obvious choice, the winner of the contest, is the person she knows will not leave, will not forsake her and will love her regardless. My job is to look beyond the anger and abuse and to live up to these unspoken expectations.

If that were the only challenge, it would be easy. The problem is that I have my own anger. I resent the cancellation of yet another vacation, the need for me to take yet another week off work to manage the house and children, the stress of holding things together and trying to comfort her at the same time. I am angry that she let it go this far. I am furious that she takes her frustration out on me. Each time she winces with pain I feel hostility, not sympathy. And as soon as the hostility wells up, it is washed away by guilt.

Anger and guilt. Guilt and anger. I don't want to burden her with the stresses in my life, so I don't tell her about the exam I failed, the patient I lost on the table or the fight I had with one of the children. If I share these stresses I feel guilty (she has enough to deal with), but if I conceal them I feel angry. I have been offered tickets to the ball game. If I go, I feel guilty, but if I decline and go to the hospital instead, I get angry. There is no escape.

Ultimately, Ferne recovers. Sometimes it's a long process involving surgery and rehabilitation, and sometimes it's only a day or two. As time goes on, we get better at communicating our anger and guilt, and although we are far from expert, we recognize and respect each other's predicament more readily than we used to. From my perspective, it's important to keep the big picture in my mind. I know that she will never be cured, and I've learned to live with that. I just keep pointing myself toward nurturing and recapturing that girl on the dock, helping her repeatedly to get back up and dust herself off, to reclaim the energy and confidence that is her essence, and to keep alive the spark that burns for both of us into the future.

EIGHTEEN

Resolution

I will never know what this life would have been like without the trials and tribulations of chronic illness. I don't know what tomorrow, next week, next year or years to come will bring for me. Some of my doctors have indicated that this disease will burn itself out and I will no longer suffer from its wrath. I hope so, but will not bet on it. Even if I become well, the many years of drug-taking and surgical interventions have altered my body beyond its innocent beginnings.

I'll never shake the feeling that one day I'll wake up and be like everyone who doesn't have to put up with the physical and emotional pain, loneliness, anger and frustration of chronic illness. I'll never stop feeling that I have suffered a loss and that this is just a bad dream.

The reality of chronic illness is that it changes your life, sometimes beyond all recognition. It's up to each of us—helpers as well as sufferers—to learn to cope with it and to incorporate new frames of reference. To learn that it can become part of your life. You can work within the framework that you have *now*, rather than fighting to find the self you have lost. If you pursue the journey for finding your old self, you will be so terribly sad to find that the old self is no longer there to be found.

Try to find new ways of defining yourself—this will be your greatest task. Once it's complete, you will be able to move forward and grow. You will take with you the experience of being in the depths of hell and surviving. You may never stop asking, "Why me?" but you will be able to answer the question. You will be able to say, "If not me, then who?" It will always feel unfair, but you will know that the height of unfairness would be to succomb to your illness.

You will have to fight long and hard to get a grip on the beginning of the climb towards coping. As each piece of rock shudders under the pressure of your footing, you will be challenged as to how far you can climb. You'll suffer setbacks and want to give up. You'll get tired and hungry for a normal life. There will even be days when you have to coax your feet to move forward, one at a time.

Ultimately, the day will arrive when you'll be able to see the beauty around you without having to first reference your illness. On that day, you will have stared hope in the face and it will have returned your stare. You will be able to find the strength to help yourself and others. This does not mean that you will never find yourself at the bottom of the mountain again. The next time, you will know the shortcuts and the routes that make the climb a little easier. Use those paths. Commit them to memory. It's your life to live. It's your responsibility to yourself and those who love you to do it to the best of your ability, now and always. If you take on this challenge, you will be rewarded with a new life. You were the captain of your destiny as much as was humanly possible. You cannot feel defeated, because you gave it your best. This new life may not resemble the one you had planned for yourself, but it will be filled with the realization that you survived. And this, in itself, will be your personal triumph.

Appendix I: A Mother's Perspective

I always knew that my mother and father had suffered with me every step of the way. Phone calls late into the night to request their help, yet again, were increasingly difficult to make. I could only guess the feelings that washed over parents each time their child's illness reared its head.

Children are always children to their parents, even when their age tells us they are adults. Parents can be torn apart by worry even when their forty-year-old child is ill. Parents always worry. So I asked Marilyn to tell me her story and I am passing it on to you.

Parenting is difficult enough and we learn as we go along. How did I know what I was doing? No one can prepare you for your child's illness. The sheer hopelessness and frustration at seeing your child suffer is almost impossible to describe. When we were confronted with a second chronically ill child, we were shocked. We muddled through, and somehow we coped. We are still learning how to cope.

In 1973, my thirteen-year-old son David, who had been a strapping, healthy child, became sickly and emaciated. My husband and I were convinced that this was more than a flu or virus. After three frustrating years of consultations and lengthy hospital stays, he was finally diagnosed with Crohn's disease. Now we had a name. I went to the local library clutching my scrap of paper with the words "Crohn's disease" written on it. I found one whole paragraph describing this illness that was ravaging my son's body.

Treatment began. David seemed to be the guinea pig for every new medication and procedure available. Most of what was tried was experimental. TPN, Imuran and prednisone were all in their infancy as treatments. David's TPN tubes kept splitting and breaking because they couldn't withstand the pressure. Blood would spurt in every direction and I would run to the nursing station in a panic—it was becoming routine. The nurses and doctors were often stymied. Strangely, David was usually the calmest of us all. He would merely clamp the spurting tube and wait for help. (He actually learned to sleep with his hand on the clamp until many years later when the technology improved.)

When mistakes were made and David suffered, we got angry. On one occasion, he received a drug he was allergic to, turned red, bruised and broke out in huge itchy lumps. We spent the next forty-eight hours bathing him every half hour. My husband was so angry he threatened to wrap David in a blanket and take him home. We felt helpless.

One of the hardest things for me was when David would apologize for being sick. He sensed our constant anguish, our guilt about being away from the other kids at home, our constant struggle to create a semblance of a "normal" family environment. Though we tried to assure him that it was no one's fault, that he would get better, that everything would improve and that we loved him, he had a tough time believing us. We had a tough time believing it ourselves.

We sought counseling and, lo and behold, it helped. We learned that every family is like a picture puzzle: if you move one piece, everything and everyone shifts. We needed to get acquainted with our new picture—we needed to learn how to cope with continual shifting. It was hard.

We decided that, no matter what, we would always treat David as normally as possible. When he was home, David was treated like everyone else. We let David judge how he felt. If he had just been released from hospital and asked to go to camp, we would breathe deeply and then calmly say, "Yes." That was tough but we put our faith in David's good judgment and our love. We didn't want to treat him differently but were never sure if we were being too harsh or too lenient. Many nights I cried myself to sleep wondering if I was doing it right.

My husband and I decided that we would always try to have one of us home at mealtimes. It was difficult, but somehow we managed. I must have put a million miles on my car. But it worked. Whenever David went into remission, we could do things together as a family— these were wonderful times. Then the illness would strike again.

When our other son Gary was diagnosed, ten years later at the age of twelve, he presented different symptoms. He remembered David's bad times and knew the prognosis as well as we did. We couldn't be optimistic about his getting better.

Gary withdrew into himself. David had always, for the most part, communicated with us. Getting used to Gary's method of coping was a new challenge. We had to learn that each child handles things differently.

In April 1974, my husband Al and I got tired of feeling lonely, angry and isolated by this illness. We appealed to other parents who were as frustrated as we were, and agreed to do some constructive handwringing: The Crohn's and Colitis Foundation of Canada (CCFC) was born. (Until recently, it was known as the Canadian Foundation for Ileitis and Colitis.) We wanted to go beyond the old adage misery loves company. We never wanted our families or our children to feel alone in this fight.

When the countless phone calls began, we were well-equipped to empathize with other people's feelings of guilt and frustration. Sharing, supporting, hand-holding, crying, learning have shown me over and over that, though details may vary, the overall feelings are the same.

"Adam doesn't want to go to school"; "my daughter refuses to talk to us"; "My son has threatened suicide"; and so on. It was never easy listening to yet another family in pain and it wan't easy to revive those familiar feelings of fear, as we listened. I would share some of my experiences, hoping it would help, and would encourage families to learn about the physical plan of their son or daughter's school. When the doors were removed from toilet stalls in high schools because of drugs, I went to the principal, requesting permission for David to use the bathroom in the teacher's lounge. Children should not be penalized for being sick. When they aren't well enough to write exams or tests, arm yourself with brochures from your local office of the CCFC or CCFA (the Crohn's and Colitis Foundation of America). Talk to the teachers, principal, nurse and other support staff. Increase their knowledge of the disease and their empathy for your child.

I have lost count of the number of procedures, surgeries and hospitalizations we have endured. Who would want to keep tabs on that? Let me tell you this. It never gets easier. The phone calls pulling us out of bed are as frightening today as they were twenty-three years ago. Some things have changed. First of all, if we are called, it's to help take care of our baby granddaughter so David's wife can take him to the hospital. Yes, David is married now. He is a physician (no, not a gastroenterologist) and has a beautiful wife and a healthy baby girl. Gary is articling for a local law firm. Both are in remission at the moment, but at the time you are reading this, who knows. I hold them up as role models and, although my maternal pride gets in the way of a true picture of my boys, I know I have every reason to be proud.

There are no easy answers. As I travel around the country, I am convinced that parents of children with Crohn's disease need to find one another. The local chapters of the CCFC and the CCFA should be able to help. We need to know about ongoing medical research and how close we are to finding the cause and cure for this awful illness. Great progress has been made in the last twenty-five years, not only medically but in the quality of life for our sons and daughters.

If I had to sum it all up, I would say, "Never, ever, lose faith." It's often one step forward and two steps back. You force yourself to feel positive when you can hardly get up and put one foot in front of the other. You force yourself to be optimistic because what else can you do? Your children will pick up on your attitude and know that if you can be positive, strong, optimistic and full of faith, so can they. Never underestimate your child. He or she can read you loud and clear, even when you don't utter a sound. You can give your children a good attitude, warm physical and emotional support, but the most important thing is unconditional love.

Marilyn's story is unique. Not everyone has two children with the same chronic illness, and not all families are open enough to seek help when they can't figure out what to do. Furthermore, not every family has two loving parents with a strong commitment to treat all members of the family equally. But many families share similarities with Marilyn's, and all families can use help coping. The next time you are in your doctor's waiting room, try to connect with the family next to you. Ask the receptionist or nurse if there is an experienced family who could help you through this experience. Call your local CCFC or CCFA and ask about a parent/child support group. You are not alone.

Appendix II: You are what you eat . . . not!

Diet shmiet—just let me eat what I want.

Okay, so most of us love ice cream sundaes, caesar salad and popcorn, mushrooms and corn on the cob. I love all these things but they don't love me. Too bad, so sad. What is a person to do?

No one seems to understand what it is like to be a person with inflammatory bowel disease trying to cope with the dietary restrictions that it brings. Much of what I am going to tell you could be stated by *anyone* who has a chronic illness. You see, it's all about food . . . aaand it isn't.

Let's back up a little. When you meet someone, and want to get to know them, what is the first thing they want to do? It's the "Lets go out for coffee, dinner, lunch, brunch" suggestion: hardly a possibility for someone on enteral feedings, home TPN or even major food intolerance of the dreaded flare-up.

Most cultures interact around food.
If you are going to celebrate a
birthday,
anniversary,
birth or promotion,
commiserate over losing a boyfriend,
girlfriend, losing your job,
Thanksgiving, football games,
hot dogs at the baseball games,
no matter what we do—our culture has us socializing around food.
When someone is sick we send them food to get well.
Food is supposed to nurture, cure, and help. It's supposed to make people feel happier if they are happy and chase the blues away if they are down.
If this is true, then you know why life feels so difficult in a world where many things have **off limits** signs.
Don't touch that chocolate sundae,
box of popcorn,
veggie and dip plate,
because, if you do . . . you might spend the rest of the night locked in the bathroom, or worse still, end up in the emergency room with a bowel obstruction. You might enjoy the taste now, but boy, will you pay later. I really hate that feeling.
You have talked about your restrictions with your dietician, you know that you shouldn't eat it but the diet you are allowed to eat is boring. Nothing seems to interest you **except the chocolate sundae**. You are caught between your rational mind and your emotional one. Anyone with food restrictions feels this way. But not everyone with food restrictions feels cheated out of control in many parts of their life.

People who have IBD and other chronic illnesses have lost control of their relationships, their daily activities, their ability to predict how they will feel next week, next month, even in the next ten minutes. Losing control of what you can eat is the last straw. A restricted diet is something that has to be dealt with at least three times a day—breakfast, lunch and dinner.

After every major surgery, I have lost many pounds, making my loved ones—and professionals—quite nervous. We do the same dance each time.

"Eat!"

"I don't want to."

"You have to."

"No, I am not hungry."

"You will get sicker."

"You won't get better." Now I feel guilty because I have the power to open my mouth and just place those calories calmly inside, but I don't. Trying to get back your appetite after a bout of illness can be difficult.

So where does that leave you? Learn to EDUCATE yourself. This does not mean to simply follow the boring diet and drone on about what you can't eat. After all, there are those people out there who claim to want to have this illness. They are the people in the crowd who would like our disease "for a week or two so they can shed those extra pounds" they put on on their last vacation or during a holiday binge. When someone says something like that to me I say, "Listen honey, if I give you this disease there is no way I am taking it back. You can have it, weight loss and all."

Try going to your local health food store or specialty

food shop and talk to the people who work there about food alternatives. They often work with people with food allergies and are happy to introduce you to a whole new world of foods you never knew existed. Be on the lookout for those high prices. Choose carefully, one new thing at a time.

The CCFC and the CCFA have free publications that focus on these issues. Call and ask for copies.

Educate the people around you. Teach them how to approach your diet. You are and generally always will be the best person to inform others of how you would like to see something handled. This holds true for your diet. I personally don't like the focus on my plate so I stick with things that don't cause problems *unless I am cheating*.

Since I am the chief cook and bottle-washer at our home, this makes the food preparation, with-restrictions-in-mind, easier. I try to remember how important those cute little calories are, especially when I am sick. If you are the chef, and don't have the disease, aiming for a meal that is as normal as possible usually works the best.

What rhymes with educate? CREATE. Be as creative as possible about the diet. Remember that your goal is to be as healthy as possible. There are cookbooks available which can help you in the right direction (please see the Recommended Reading list). Go to your local bookstore and spend some time in the food section. Jewish kosher cookbooks use a lot of milk substitutes for people who have lactose intolerance. Low-fat cooking, all the rage, helps those of us who have difficulty digesting fat. This requires research and a trip out, but the results are worth it.

I will share a trade secret with you. When you are feeling down, take yourself to the grocery store, either physically (which is optimal) or mentally, by visualizing the trip. Satisfy your cravings. Purchase a small amount of anything you think you might want to eat and indulge in. Did you have a "comfort" food before you got sick? Not everything has to be good for you.

People with severe food restrictions can play around with their taste buds with various fruit candies, Jell-O, soup or lollipops. Make sure you check with your physician first. The way the food is presented is the key. Whether it is on a stick, in a bowl or on a plate, all affect how good it will look to you. Even a can of food-supplement served in a frosty soda-fountain glass can seem appealing. After all, everything is packaging. Ask any disappointed five year old, after she discovers the breakfast cereal that her mom brought home from the store doesn't really dance around and leap out of the bowl to play with her.

Lastly, you must learn to COMMUNICATE. Restaurants and dinner-party invitations can be problematic. For restaurants, call ahead and check out the menu before you go. Most places have a wide enough variety to satisfy most restrictions. For dinner parties, I will often offer to bring something, to ensure that there is a safe dish for me to eat. If my host asks if she can make a meal— being considerate of my food restrictions—I always say no. Why? Because when I allow the menu to be tailored to my restrictions, the dinner conversation turns to my restricted diet and IBD, which is something I would prefer to play down.

Remember, it is **your** approach to your diet that is the

key. Get in touch with how you feel about food and about life in general with food restrictions? Take a moment to try on some of what I have told you. Remember to ED-UCATE yourself, be CREATIVE, and COMMUNI-CATE with others. Can you do it? Of course you can.

Glossary of Medical Terminology

Barium—a fine, milky liquid that is used as a contrast medium in X-rays of the bowel. The movement of barium is followed by fluoroscopy and X-ray studies to look for and diagnose conditions of the esophagus, stomach and intestinal tract.

Breath Test—these tests are currently being used to diagnose lactose malabsorption and bacterial overgrowth. After swallowing a test substance, the patient (over the next few hours) periodically breathes into a tube attached to a container. The test is simple and painless but the drink tastes somewhat yucky.

Bowel Rest—through the use of either oral elemental diets or intravenous nutrition, the bowel is given a rest by not having to digest any food. This time allows the bowel to heal.

Castor Oil—an oily preparation used for constipation and cleansing the bowel or colon before an examination. (Mix in orange juice and plug your nose.)

Cecum—the first portion of the large bowel; one end is attached to the ileum.

Central Venous Catheter—a hollow flexible tube that is inserted into the subclavian vein to give total parenteral nutrition.

Chronic Illness—a disease that usually develops slowly but persists for a long time, often for the remainder of the person's lifetime.

Colitis—an inflammation of the large bowel; affected areas of the colon can lose the smooth lining, bleed more easily and develop ulcers.

Colon—the large bowel, which receives waste products from the ileum, or last portion of the small intestine, and is responsible for the absorption of water from the feces; solid stool is then delivered into the rectum prior to a bowel movement.

Colonoscopy—a mildly uncomfortable but extremely useful diagnostic procedure in which a fiberoptic tube is inserted into the rectum and then advanced into the cecum in order to visualize the lining of the entire colon. It is useful for obtaining biopsies and removing polyps.

Crohn's Disease—a chronic inflammatory bowel disease of unknown origin that can affect any part of the gastro-intestinal tract but most commonly the ileum and colon. It is characterized by frequent attacks of diarrhea, severe abdominal pain, nausea, fever, chills, weakness, anorexia and weight loss.

Distended—swollen; often refers the the bowel or bladder.

Duodenum—the first part of the small intestine immediately after the stomach.

Elemental Diets—synthetic powder or liquid preparations that contain all essential nutrients to sustain the body. These are absorbed easily by the bowel and are taken orally (they usually have an unpleasant taste) or by nasogastric tube.

Endoscopy—a procedure in which a fiberoptic instrument is swallowed by a heavily sedated patient to visualize portions of the intestine. A gastroscopy is an endoscopy of the esophagus, stomach and duodenum; a colonoscopy is an endoscopy of the colon.

Enteritis—an inflammaton of the small intestine.

ET (Enterostomal Therapist)—a registered nurse who has been specially trained in the physical and emotional support of patients with stomas. These include bowel as well as urinary diversions.

Exacerbation—an increase in the seriousness of a disease, which is shown by the signs or symptoms of the patient growing worse.

Gastroenterologist—a physician who specializes in the study of diseases affecting the gastrointestinal tract, which includes the esophagus, stomach, intestines, gall bladder and bile duct.

GI Series (Gastrointestinal Series)—a series of X-rays that examine and lend information to the diagnosis of gastrointestinal diseases. These usually include a Barium swallow or small bowel enema to examine the upper GI tract, and a barium enema to examine the lower bowel.

IBD—Inflammatory Bowel Disease.

Ileitis—an inflammation of the ileum, common in Crohn's disease patients.

Ileostomy—a surgically created opening in the abdominal wall. A loop of bowel is brought to the surface of the abdomen and sutured in place. A disposable bag is placed over the piece of bowel (stoma). This bag is emptied into the toilet four to six times each day. The person has no control over the movement of his or her bowels.

Ileum—the lower two-fifths of the small intestine.

Imuran—an immuno-suppressive drug that prevents the body's immune system from reacting to the disease or an environmental agent.

Intravenous (IV)—an infusion set that includes a glass bottle or a plastic bag containing fluid or nutrients connected to a catheter or a needle in the patient's vein.

Jejunum—the upper third of the small intestine.

Kock Ileostomy—a new surgical procedure; this type of ileostomy is performed on patients with ulcerative colitis (no external bag is required—the patient empties the reservoir at appropriate intervals).

Lactose Intolerance—a sensitivity disorder of the body caused by the absence of the enzyme lactase, which causes an inability to digest lactose, a sugar found in milk products. Symptoms are bloating, gas, nausea, diarrhea and abdominal cramps.

Mononucleosis—a viral illness caused by the Epstein-Barr virus and characterized by fever, sore throat, swollen lymph glands, enlarged liver and spleen and severe fatigue.

Nasogastric Tube—a tube that is placed through the nose into the stomach to relieve gastric distension. It is also used to administer elemental diets for patients on bowel rest.

Percussion (percussed)—a technique in physical examination performed by striking the fingers, in which the size, borders and consistency of internal organs are determined.

Perforation—an abnormal opening in the wall of the bowel when an area of the bowel becomes weakened; contents of the bowel spill into the abdominal cavity.

Perianal—an irritation or inflammation around the anus common to patients with inflammatory bowel syndrome, particularly those with Crohn's disease.

Peritonitis—an inflammation of the membrane that covers the entire abdominal wall of the body. This is a medical emergency and the patient is in severe pain.

Polyp—a growth that protrudes into the intestinal tube and which can be removed at the time of colonoscopy; some are due to inflammation (pseudo-polyps) and others are real growths.

Post-operative Pneumonia—a form of pneumonia that is caused by reduced expansion of the lung due to pain and inadequate mobilization.

Prednisone—an anti-inflammatory drug prescribed for severe inflammation and immuno-suppression.

Pyoderma Gangrenosum—a rare type of skin sore that can occur on the legs of patients with ulcerative colitis or Crohn's disease.

Quiescent—when a disease backs off and becomes inactive.

Rectum—the lower portion of the large bowel, connecting the sigmoid colon and the anus.

Remission—the partial or complete disappearance of the symptoms of a chronic illness or malignant disease.

Resection—indicates that a portion of the bowel has been surgically removed.

Sigmoidoscopy—a procedure using the sigmoidoscope, an instrument consisting of a tube and a light for visualization of the mucous membrane of the colon.

Stoma—an artifical opening of an internal organ on the surface of the body, created surgically as for a colostomy or ileostomy.

Total Parenteral Nutrition (TPN)—the intravenous administration of a complete diet consisting of proteins, fats and sugars. The solution is irritating to the veins and is usually given through a central venous catheter.

Triage—a process in which a group of patients is sorted according to their need for care. The severity of the problem governs the process.

Typhoid Fever—a bacterial infection characterized by headache, delirium, watery diarrhea, cough, rash and high fever.

Toxic Megacolon—a serious complication of ulcerative colitis or Crohn's disease that may result in perforation of the colon, severe blood infection (septicemia) and death. Surgery is the usual treatment.

Ulcer (Duodenal)—a crater-like lesion of the lining of the duodenum that results from inflammation or infection.

Ultrasound—an abdominal ultrasound, instead of an X-ray, is commonly done on patients with IBD. An ultrasound, which uses sound waves to visualize different parts of the body, can visualize the liver, gall bladder, bowel ducts and pancreas, as well as kidneys.

Upper GI Series—an X-ray of the esophagus, stomach and duodenum after the ingestion of liquid barium.

Recommended Reading

Understanding the Disease

Banks, P.A., D.H. Present and P. Steiner. *The Crohn's Disease and Ulcerative Colitis Fact Book*. New York: Charles Scribner's Sons, 1983.

Brandt, L. and P. Steiner-Grossman. *Treating IBD: A Patient's Guide to the Medical and Surgical Management of Inflammatory Bowel Disease*. New York: Raven Press, 1989.

Korelitz, B., Sohn, N. *Inflammatory Bowel Disease, Experience and Controversy*. Florida: Grune & Stratton, Inc., 1985. Gawain, S. Creative Visualization. Toronto: Bantam New Age Book, 1985.

Steiner, P., P.A. Banks and D.H. Present. *People . . . Not Patients: A Source Book for Living With Inflammatory Bowel Disease*. New York: National Foundation for Ileitis and Colitis, 1991.

Thompson, W.G. *The Angry Gut: Coping With Colitis and Crohn's Disease*. New York: Plenum Publishing, 1993.

"Living With" Issues

Kron, Audrey. *Ask Audrey*. Michigan: Centre for Coping With Chronic Illness (810-626-6960), 1992.

Krauss, P. *Why Me? Coping With Grief, Loss and Change*. New York: Bantam Books, 1988.

Kubler-Ross, E. *On Death and Dying*. New York: Macmillan Publishing Company, 1974.

Kushner, H. *When All You've Ever Wanted Isn't Enough: The Search for a Life That Matters*. New York: Summit Books, 1986.

*Kushner, H. *When Bad Things Happen to Good People*. New York: Avon, 1983.

*LeMaistre, J. *Beyond Rage*. Palo Alto: Alpine Guild, 1985.

Nielsen, P. *Will of Iron*. Ann Arbor: Momemtum Books, 1992.

Pitzele, Sefra. *We Are Not Alone*. New York: Workman Publishing, 1986.

*Quindlen, A. *Living Out Loud*. New York: IVY Books, 1988.

Register, C. *Living With Chronic Illness: Days of Patience and Passion*. New York: The Free Press, 1987.

Samuels, Rebecca. *When Mommy Gets Sick*. LFA Inc., 4 Research Place, Suite 180, Rockville MD: 1992.

*Siegal, Bernie. *Love, Medicine and Miracles*. New York: Harper & Row, 1986.

Siegal, Bernie. *Peace, Love and Healing*. New York: HarperPerennial, 1989.

Siegal, M. and P. Donoghue. *Sick of Feeling Tired*. New York: W.W. Norton & Company, 1993.

Skilken, P.S. *Never Apologize, Always Explain*. New York : Everest House, 1982.

Sontag, S. *Illness as Metaphor*. New York: Farrar Straus & Giroux,1978

Stearns, Ann Kaiser. *Coming Back*. New York: Random House,1988.

*Strong, M. *Mainstay: For the Well Spouse of the Chronically Ill*. Boston: Little Brown and Company, 1988.

Nutrition and Diet

Greenwood, Jan K. *The IBD Nutrition Book*. New York: John Wiley & Sons, 1992.

Scanlon, Deralee. *The Wellness Book of IBD*. New York: St. Martins Press, 1989.

Waisman, Mary Sue. *A Special Kind of Cookbook*. Manitoba: Derksen Printers Ltd., 1989

*Ferne's favorites